Memoirs of a Student

Memoirs of a Student

Professional associates of author

Dr. Roscoe Arnold Dykman

.

For Medical Sciences (1955-2014)
Student University of Arkansas (Math Dept. 2012)
Memoirs of a Student

Roscoe A. Ryman, Ph. D
Professor Emeritus
University of Arkansas

Abstract

———— ❧ ————

THIS PAPER COVERS much of the research completed by collaborators and myself. It lists stepwise people who inspired me, and whom I came to know through Dr. Gantt, the last American to work with Pavlov, and his scientific and literary friends. It includes Pavlov's outstanding student Saroyan, and Dos Passas, Scott Fitzgerald, Bernard Shaw, and many others. Excepting Dos Passos, most of Gantt's literary friends were deceased when I joined Gantt at Hopkins in 1950. I learned about these friends through taped interviews we made with Dr. Gantt. My four main professors at the University of Chicago were Kleitman, Havighurst, Rogers, and Krogman. These teachers including Gantt influenced nearly everything that I and my associates published. The validity of the comments of prominent others Hebb, Lorenz, Skinner, Shaw, not supportive of Russian research on the underlying theory of the conditional reflex, influenced the criticisms Gantt and Pavlov made of American psychology. A theme that runs through much of this account is whether Russian research with its anti-statistical bias, and emphasis upon the biological basis of the conditional reflexes, or ecological research, which favors instinctive theory, or operant conditioning, which ignores biological causation, should be included under the single heading conditional reflex. Hilgard and Marquis (1940) described Pavlov's, conditioning studies as classical to distinguish it from other kinds of conditioning. However, Pavlov and Gantt did operant experiments, but less complicated than the variable ratio schedules that Dr. Marr (2011) describes in a paper, which describes the methods he employed to teach children with both ADHD and reading disorders to ignore distractions. However, both Pavlov and Gantt would have described these clever experiments as conditional reflexes.

Two people played an important role in the development of this manuscript. The first was Mallory Nash, a graduate student of the University of Arkansas, who helped with all the typing after it was translated using Dragon. The second was Jack Marr, professor of Psychology at the University of Arkansas, who looked at an earlier version of the manuscript and made suggestions.

Background

―――――― ❦ ――――――

THE PAIRING OF a conditional stimulus (CS) with an unconditional stimulus (UCS), such as electrical stimulation or food, produces conditional reflexes (CRs) in multiple organ systems. Most studies report-conditioning results for only 1-4 organs (often only one). Physiologists working in laboratories across the hall from mine at Hopkins thought it would be impossible to condition responses mediated by the autonomic nervous system (ANS). They based their reasoning upon mechanisms of homeostasis described in physiological texts written in the 1940s and 50s. An experiment described below, indicated that they were wrong (Dykman, Corson, Reese, & Seager, 1962). Gantt's research is explained by verbal constructs he had developed 40 years before I joined him in 1950. We used his concepts to explain our research that Gantt had developed over the past 40 years from research on autonomic and motor conditioning. These include the homeostatic processes regulating organ system responsibility; schizokinesis which often overrides homeostatic mechanisms to produce new and unexpected CRs; autokinesis which describes pathological behaviors that develop over time, following experiences such as starvation or pain. These also appear in n animals and humans who overreact to everyday stresses of life. Hence, the term conditional reflex has a much broader meaning than that of classical conditioning. However, they did not know or believe that the pairing of stimulus was more powerful than the linear pairing of the CS with the UCS.

All of my life, I have been rewarded by propinquity - right time, place, and people. I never applied for an academic position. Job offers were just happy events. About the time I was finishing my academic work at the University of Chicago, I was looking for a thesis project. At that time, I was taking a course in physiological psychology taught by Tom Andrews, an

Assistant Professor in the Psychology Department. He described the research that Phil Shurrager had completed on spinal conditioning, saying that he was Chairman of the Department of Psychology at Illinois Institute of Technology (IIT), a very good engineering school. In concluding his lecture on spinal conditioning, Andrews said that most psychologists working in the area of classical conditioning did not regard the Shurrager study as true conditioning. Kellogg (1946) and many others argued that Shurrager's spinal conditioning should be interpreted as sensitization rather than conditioning.

I needed a thesis project, and the possibility of spinal conditioning with its implications for spinal cord injuries appealed to me. I called Dr. Shurrager and arranged a visit. He was happy to see me, and after a lengthy interview, he offered me a job as an Instructor, which I quickly accepted. I did my doctoral studies in his laboratory while teaching most of the introductory courses in psychology offered at IIT, and auditing all the undergraduate courses in math, including linear algebra at night, a course needed for an understanding of factor analysis. The latter was a work in progress that I continued for several years after I moved to other jobs.

Dr. Robrrt J. Havighurst (1900-1991)

I was already a student at Chicago when I met Dr. Shurrager. Of the famous person's I met or worked with, Dr. Havighurst did more for me than anyone else by admitting me as a graduate student in Human Development at the University of Chicago (1946-1949). I can honestly say it was a touch and go situation for a while, and it all occurred after I had come back from World War II to complete one year of college. Grades in my sophomore year at Idaho State University (then Southern Branch) were well below those expected for University of Chicago applicants. I was dating my wife to be, and my spare time was occupied by dating. I was also on the track team, teaching swimming at the local YMCA, and earning money for tuition and books. I left Idaho State University in 1941 to enter George Williams College, one of two very good schools that educated physical directors and executives for YMCA jobs. Except for one misguided academic year, I was a good student, graduating with the highest grades in my class from George Williams College in 1946, and winning the Earl Eubank Scholarship Award. After some goading from my undergraduate college president at George Williams College, Havighurst decided to let me take the University graduate reading examination. Fortunately, the test score was sufficient for admittance to University of Chicago.

Dr. Havighurst developed a list of developmental tasks normally achieved at different age levels. This became the basis for the future development of many psychological tests assessing the development of children, teenagers, and adults. The third edition of his well-known book on human growth was entitled, "*Developmental Tasks and Education* (1972)."

Dr. Havighurst's father and mother were on the faculty at Lawrence College, and they placed him in prep schools where he won many awards for scholarship. He had a Ph.D. in physics, and I asked him on one of my frequent visits, why he gave up a prestigious field such as physics for human development, and he said, "I thought human development was more important." He had published a number of papers in Physics and Chemistry Journals on the structure of the atom. His education included honors and awards from many schools (Ohio State University, 1924, Ph.D. in Chemistry and Physics, and Fulbright scholar University of Canterbury, New Zealand, 1961). He entered the field of human development in 1928, and became a Professor of Education at the University of Chicago, and Chairman of the University Committee on Human Development. I was attracted to the diversity of the curriculum of human development; it allowed students to take for credit or audit almost any course taught by the University, while taking the core courses in human development.

My background in biology interested Dr. Havighurst. He knew my professor of physiology at George Williams College, Dr. Arthur Steinhaus (1897-1970), who received all of his college degrees from the University of Chicago. Dr. Steinhaus was a well-known expert in physical fitness and sports. He was the best teacher I ever had in terms of interpreting the facts of physiology. He was very much opposed to boxing as a sport that damaged the brain. I was frightened by this since I had started boxing at the age of 12, and continued this while in the army in World War II. Dr. Steinhaus was disturbed to find out I had been boxing while I was in the Army and earlier in my life. So, one night he took me to a meeting of the retired boxers living in Chicago. Every ex-boxer met exhibited conspicuous signs of brain damage such as, hand tremors, slurred speech, stuttering, balancing problems in walking or standing, and an inability to comprehend speech. Many of them were drinking alcohol, and told us horror stories about their boxing careers, and their other traumatic experiences. I often wondered how many IQ points I lost with the hits in the head.

Dr. Steinhaus encouraged me to audit medical school courses at the University of Chicago. I started out by asking the teacher of pharmacology, if he would let me audit his course. He said he would, providing I first take the course in organic chemistry for a grade. I enrolled in pharmacy my first two years at Idaho State University, and took some very good courses in chemistry, avoiding organic chemistry. As anticipated, organic chemistry turned out to be a very difficult course, but I made it through, and I then spent a semester auditing an even more difficult course, medical school pharmacology.

Because of my interest in biomedical sciences, Dr. Havighurst invited me after graduation to return to Chicago one month each year to lecture on the biology of Human Development (1949-1953). He also offered me a chance to join the University of Chicago faculty, heading a social class study of a small Midwestern town, similar in design to the study of social classes Dr. Lloyd Warner described in his book *"Yankee City"*. When Warner was a professor at Harvard, he did a study of primitive people living in the South Pacific islands. After speaking with reporters about this study, the San Francisco Examiner ran the following headline, "Harvard professor discovers love nest in the South Pacific." Warner had moved to Chicago, and I took every course he taught.

Willian Marion Krogman (1903-1987)

Dr. Krogman was a brilliant and inspiring teacher. In the physical anthropology course I took in 1946 at the University of Chicago, he spent much of his time discussing human development, and particularly the changes, which occur with age in bone structure, dentition, and behavior. We had a syllabus, but none of his popular books were required reading in this introductory course. We dissected guinea pigs and turtles to study differences in body structure with an emphasis on the structure of brains in different species. He brought human brains into class. The brains were stored in jars of formaldehyde, and sliced to reveal their 3D structures. We were required to learn the names of all the parts, and their connections with each other. I remember something Krogman said about height, "An adult dwarf was asked by a man, "Why are you so short?" The dwarf replied, "I am as big for me as you are for you."

Interestingly, even though he was a superb teacher, I found out in writing about him that I knew very little about his professional prominence, or his history. He never mentioned his intellectual accomplishments in lecturing. I learned about these from reading an excellent history, *"A Biographical Memoir by William A. Haviland"* (1994) written by William Haviland (1994), honoring his friend Bill. This article was published by the National Academy of Sciences. Haviland must have been a very good friend of Dr. Krogman, since he referred to him repeatedly as Bill. I will mention some of the highlights of his long article.

> *"Krogman's major contributions and his most important contributions were, however, in the areas of child growth and development, and forensic anthropology. The latter specialty was practically invented by Krogman in his book; "The Human Skeleton in Forensic Medicine (1962)" remains the definitive source for medical and police professionals alike. Krogman's studies are used by health professionals throughout America to evaluate the growth of children (p. 294)."*

Krogman's parents emigrated from Germany, and he grew up in Oak Park Illinois. His father was a carpenter, who built a house designed by Frank Lloyd Wright. He chose every piece of lumber that went into the construction of that house. According to Haviland, "Krugman was deeply affected by his father's rigorous standards of workmanship, and the integrity that went into his work."

Krogman said that he and his twin brother often pretended to dig for pirate treasure. On one of the digs, they uncovered the bones of a horse's head, and then continued to dig for all the bones of the horse, which was lying on its side. Krogman later said, "These youthful digs would not have been approved by modern archaeologists. Here I venture to say, was an early foray into my future studies of Comparative Anatomy and Physical Anthropology." Hence, he was off to a very good start, and this showed up in1932, when he took the entrance examination of the University of Chicago, placing first among 490 applicants. In his senior year in college, he was assigned the task of writing a term paper on the subject of physical anthropology. The paper focused upon the dentition of primates, including man. One of the reviewers of his paper, who later hired Krogman, suggested that he enter a contest. He won first prize receiving an award of $25,000, a large amount of money in 1932. I was 12 at the time, and my mother would give me a quarter to go to the store and buy salmon or pork chops. A quarter would buy six large salmon steaks or pork chops. A nickel would buy a candy bar four times larger than those that now cost more than a dollar.

Krogman secured a job as a graduate student which placed him in charge of the summer digs of the Archeological Survey of Illinois (1929-1930). He received his Ph.D. from the University of Chicago in 1930, and went on to become the chair of the National Science Foundation, and the leader of many other prominent organizations. Membership in many other onerous societies followed his retirement from the University of Chicago.

Krogman gained a reputation as a bone detective early in his academic career. He was frequently consulted by the FBI or Police when bones of humans were found in unexpected places. He was hired as a consultant in the Lindbergh kidnapping case. Krogman also was an avid Sherlock Holmes fan. He wrote several stories about Conan Doyle including one in which Holmes was portrayed as an anthropologist. He was asked to determine the age of Pharaoh Ramesses III at the time of his death. He was often asked to identify victims of violence, such as the remains of Mob Murder victims, whose bodies had been thrown into the woods of New Jersey.

Krogman was a National Research Council Fellow with Sir Arthur Keith at the Royal College of Surgeons in London. Here, he studied biostatistics with the son of Karl Pearson, who is still widely recognized for his statistical papers. The Pearson Product Moment Correlation Coefficient and Chi Square are statistics most often seen in research papers, but Pearson developed many others, useful in analyzing both quantitative and qualitative data.

Carl R. Rogers (1902-1987)

He was my favorite teacher, perhaps because I was more interested in psychology than in any other course. Rogers had a way of getting every person who became acquainted with him involved in his thinking and his understanding of behavior. He came across as a trusting, loving person. He generally opened his lectures by discussing a subject in detail he had been thinking about, and invited students to comment. He demonstrated a sincere interest in what the students had to say and often modified his own thinking by what they said. This was an opportunity for him to reinforce student's interests, making it clear that he truly appreciated their feelings and thinking. Attendance in his classes was close to 100%. You had better get to class early, if you wanted a good seat. He was always thinking of something new, which is shown by the progression of the books he wrote. Much of his history is beautifully described in an article by Kathy Jo Hall (1997).

> *"Carl R. Rogers is known as the father of client – centered therapy. Throughout his career, he dedicated himself to humanistic psychology, and he is well known for his theory of personality development. He began developing his humanistic concept while working with abused children. Rogers attempted to change the world of psychotherapy when he boldly claimed that psychoanalytic, experimental, and behavioral therapies were preventing*

their clients from ever reaching self-actualization and self-growth, due to their authoritative analysis. Rogers received wide acclaim for his studies, and was awarded various high honors. Through Rogers's extensive efforts expressing his area personality by the publishing of books and lectures, he gained a lot of attention and followers, as well as those who strongly disagreed with his theories of personality development.

Rogers was born in Oak Park Illinois in 1902. He received his B.A. from the University of Wisconsin in 1924, an M.A. from Columbia University in 1928, and his Ph.D. in psychotherapy from Columbia University in 1931. In 1940, Rogers became professor of psychology at Ohio State University where he stayed until 1945. He then transferred to the University of Chicago, here he served as a professor of psychology and the executive secretary of the Counseling Center.

Rogers has authored over 100 publications explaining his theory of personality development. He received various awards and recognitions for his contributions to the world of psychology. He received the Nicholas Murray Butler Silver Medal from Columbia University in 1955 and a special contribution award from the American Psychological Association in 1956 for his research in psychotherapy. In 1944 he was elected President of the American Association for Applied Psychology, and in 1946, was elected President of the American psychological Association." (Hall 1997).

I followed his career from the time he left Chicago, where he opened up a private clinic in California. I attended one of these sessions in which surgeons from medical schools had come because of personal problems in their lives. Their unrecognized needs to become more humanistic persons was first recognized under Roger's therapy. Rogers was able to get them just as involved in therapy, as he did with his graduate students at the University of Chicago. He moved to University of Wisconsin in 1957. I heard from a clinical psychologist there that his research methods did not match the standards expected. Whether this was true, I do not know. I was hesitant to ask him about this, when I met him in California. He apparently was at Wisconsin for about 5 years, and during his last year (1962), he served as a member of the executive Committee.

Rogers wrote three books: *"Client Centered Therapy*, (1951), *Counseling and Psychotherapy (1942)*, and *On Becoming a Person* (1961)." I have interviewed several hundred parents of children and teenagers who are hyperactive, impulsive and/or inattentive (diagnosis ADHD). I usually began the parent interviews with nondirective therapy as described by Rogers in his first book. Many married couples with hyperactive children have different opinions about the treatment of their children, particularly those regarding appropriate rewards and punishments. I liked to work with both parents at one time (not always possible). Their child or children were gradually included in the interview. After 5-10 nondirective sessions, I generally switched to meditation methods, giving parents a 'Mantra' coupled with breathing instructions. There is a much overlap in therapies whether nondirective, Gestalt, or Behavioral.

Dr. Dennis Molfese

In describing his research at Nebraska, Dr. Molfese did not discuss his previous positions as chair of Psychology at Indiana State or Louisville. I will first cite the information Dr. Molfese (Dennis to me) entered in describing his position at Nebraska. Dennis Molfese, Ph.D., is an internationally recognized expert on the use of brain recording techniques to study emerging relationships between brain development, language, and cognitive processes. Dennis received his Ph.D. in Psychology from the Pennsylvania State University. He is Chancellor's Professor Director of the Brain Imaging Center at the University of Nebraska-Lincoln, and Director of the Neuroscience Laboratory there. He is the Innovator-Editor-in-Chief for the scientific journal, Developmental Neuropsychology, and serves on the editorial boards for the Analysis of Dyslexia, and for Eye and

Brain. Dennis chairs a number of national panels in the USA, on Learning Disabilities, as well as on numerous NIB, NINH, and NSF grant review panels. He is the director of one of 15 national laboratories in the USA, which make up the National Institutes of Health, Reading and Learning Disabilities Research. He is also the recipient of a number of honors for outstanding research contributions from societies such as Sigma XI and Pi Kappa PHI. He received the Kentucky Psychologist of the Year Award, an honor most scientists would love to receive (it carries with it a substantial stipend). He is a fellow of the American Psychological Association, and the American Psychological Society. His research has been continuously funded since 1975, through grants from the National Institutes of Health, the National Science Foundation, the Department of Education, and the National Foundation for the March of Dimes, the MacArthur Foundation, Kellogg Foundation, NATO, and NASA. He has had numerous research fellows, graduate students, and technicians working in his laboratory, all highly qualified. He is a superb teacher.

In describing his research at Nebraska, Dennis did not discuss his previous positions as Chairman of Psychology at Indiana State or Louisville. As I recall, I worked with him from 2004 to 2009. It was one of the most enjoyable experiences of my life. The paper he and colleagues wrote in the book edited by Pisoi and Remez (2005) describes his Event Related Potential (ERP) research, which Dennis is continuing at Nebraska. Many difficult problems are encountered in the accurate recording of ERP's. Dennis knows as much about ERP research as anyone in the US or elsewhere, and has solved the most important problems. I also learned much about statistical data processing working on research Dennis had collected over the years.

I remember him saying when I told him that he was the last person I worked with before I completely retired, and he facetiously said, "Well you saved the best for last." I first met Dennis at a meeting of the Psychophysiological Society about 1950, and that was the start of an instantaneous friendship. I was 30 years old at the time, and had just written an NIH proposal for a fellowship at Hopkins. He was, as I recall, the

Chairman of the Psychology Department at Indiana State at that time, and was seeking research support from NIH. This was a number of years before he did very important baby research, showing that babies who are excellent in language processing skills at birth had better grades in school at the age of 8 than those deficient in differentiating differences in the sounds of letters. I shall always remember the excellent reviews he made of research proposals, which contributed to his successful career in Developmental Psychology at NIH (he and I were on some of the same NIH committees for a number of years). The journal he developed, and continues to edit, Developmental Neuropsychology contains articles in every issue, relevant to brain development, including one I wrote on the effects of nutrition on brain development. He now has equipment at Nebraska enabling him to record separately or together fMRI, MRI, and ERPs. I doubt that there are any laboratories in the U.S. as flexible and well-equipped as his.

He gave me a copy of the book by Pistoni and Remez saying, "Thanks for your friendship, guidance, and humor." This was really appreciated, but in no way equals the things he did for me, or the support he gave to Peggy Ackerman and other members of my staff, when I was chairman of the Brain Developmental Laboratory at Arkansas Children's Hospital. He came as a participant in many site visits we had from USAG-ARS (United States Department of Agriculture). We had a continuous supply of research money from 1950 to 2004, attributable in large part to the collaboration of Peggy Ackerman, other persons on my staff, and Dennis.

Psychophysiological Studies

The reader may be very confused by the physiological results of this paper. Now it is clear, that skin resistance responds to the order of stimuli. If a tone is followed by an emotional experience, the tone is dominant. If the emotional experience occurs first, it is dominant. If both occur together, the emotional experience dominates. Heartrate and respiration are monitored without any stimulation. Heartrate is perfectly correlated with respiration, with correlation coefficients exceeding .90. This means over 90% of the scatter of the responses (variance) is explained. When you scale the responses by dividing by their scatter (standard deviations), it turns out heartrate determines the respiratory rate and not the reverse. Apparently, breathing depends on changes in heartrate, not on respiration.

Figure 1 shows the stimulant medication that was most commonly used for the treatment of impulsive and hyperactive children at the time we did the study. It is often used now in combination with other stimulant drugs, which have been proven to be more efficient than methylphenidate. It remains the choice of drugs for many pediatricians. Stimulant drugs influence a very important "feel-good" neurotransmitter, dopamine, which has been shown to be deficient in hyperactive-impulsive children. The lines in Figure 1 are statically significant, and show variables that affect the amount of methylphenidate given to children at the time of the study. Drug trials usually begin with a very low dose, and the amount administered is slowly increased, if necessary, until a level is reached that ameliorates symptoms that interfere with the child's progress in school. Dose adjustments generally go on for several months or even several years. The number of children studied varied from 20 to 159 boys in different investigations. In one study (Dykman and Ackerman, 1993 chapter in a book edited by Johny Matson), we tested 58 Non-Dyslexic boys and 64 Dyslexic Boys, assigned to categories on the basis of their scores in reading. They were classified into six groups: only attention problems (Attention Deficit Disorder, (ADD), ADD +Hyperactivity, and ADD + Hyperactivity + Aggressive Behavior. We also studied these same categories of behavior in 64 boys who were dyslexic (poor readers). We will not summarize all findings her. The Yale Scale of ADHD has a category named Emotionality (Shaywitz, 1979). We used this measure to look at the relation of emotion to the other categories just described above. As was expected, higher scores in emotional behavior was associated with higher scores in all six categories listed above, except for the ADHD. The combined effect of all the variables in figure 1, assessed via multiple correlation, indicated that the variables taken together explained 90% of the variance in drug dosage.

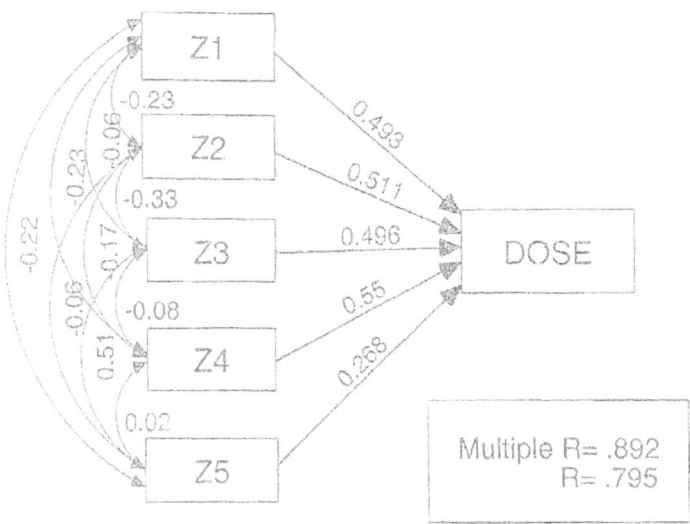

Figure 1 Multiple regression analysis predicting methylphenidate dosage levels from five sets of variables. Z1 = age + weight, Z2 = ERP type – reaction time(RT) slope, Z3 = press RT low reward – press RT no reward, Z4 =3 x heart rate (HR) high reward + HR low reward 2 x HR no reward, Z5 = skin conductance counts low reward – 2 x SC counts high reward. *See text for discussion.*

We next studied intersession adaptation and intersession extinction of the orienting response (OR). The paper describes the equipment used to monitor physiological processes, providing definitions of variables used by Gal Brecht, Dykman, Reese, & Suzuki, 1965. Research on the orienting response (OR) was stimulated by the research of Sokolov (1960, 1963). Sokolov (1960) defined the OR as a response induced by any novelty in the environment. He assumed that the (OR) was nonspecific as regards modality, the intensity of the stimulus, including both adaptation and extinction. He said that the OR should not be confused with two other types of unconditional reflexes; the adaptive and defensive reflexes (Sokolov, 1960, p. 189). He had found that the first few presentations of warmth dilated the blood vessels of the head while constricting the vessels of the finger, the latter pattern presumably common to a great variety of novel stimuli. Pavlov previously described the OR as an investigatory reflex. He wrote as follows:

> "I call it the 'What is it' reflex? This reflex brings about an immediate response in Man and animals to the slightest change in the world around, so they immediately orientate their appropriate receptor organs in accordance with the perceptible quality of the stimulus, in the agent instigating the change, making full investigation of it. The biological significance of this reflex is obvious. If the animal were not provided with, such a reflex, its life would hang it every moment by a thread. In Man, this reflex is been greatly developed with far-reaching results, being represented in the highest form by inquisitiveness - the parent of that scientific method through which we may hope someday to come to true orientation and knowledge of the world around us" (in Anrep's 1960 translation of Pavlov, p.12).

Sokolov studied only some components of the OR, and it remains to be seen whether different orienting stimuli have the common effects he assumed. We expect that studies involving a reasonable sample of bodily functions will reveal important differences between ORs to visual and auditory stimuli. It is important to discriminate between general bodily effects such as changes in heart rate (HR), respiratory rate (RR), skin resistance (SR), and muscle action potentials (MPs), from more specific bodily effects such as gastrointestinal secretions to a specific food, flexion to galvanic stimulation, vasodilation to dilation to warmth, and motor orienting reactions. The best way to do this is to classify reactions, as Sokolov does, on the basis their generality or specificity to different stimuli. This should exclude incentive and noxious stimuli (food and electrical stimulation). Also, the definition of the OR should include only those components that appear reliably on the first presentation of a novel stimulus. These components should exhibit variation within and across organ systems.

Non-reinforced tones increase HR in dogs, but rarely do so in humans. In fact, the human HR response to a novel stimulus is deceleration (Dykman and Gantt, 1959). It is important to realize that the OR is both a protective reflex and at the same time a very dangerous reflex. Hunters stop rabbits from running by whistling, making them an easy target. Any stimulus, which initiates investigation, has the potential to be harmful. From our point of view, the OR is a gross organismic response consisting of components that vary with the nature of stimuli, and within and between species.

A number of American investigators studied the OR, or the equivalent reactions under other names (Darrow, 1929). Two studies indicate that the SR component of the OR habituates by the fifth trial (Betterment & Holtzmann, 1952) and (Howe, 1958). Spontaneous recovery of the SR component is also been shown in a test-retest situation with faster habituation during recordings made at rest 6-8 weeks after the initial habituation (Rahman, 1960). In one of the earlier studies, Davis, Buchwald & Fankmann, (1955) reported effects of trials and different intensities of stimuli. Davis (1953) and Davis (1955) showed habituation gradients for muscle action potentials (MPs). The MPs had a shorter latency than the OR (200 to 300 msec.), suggesting that the OR was preceded by the startle reflex.

Dykman, Reese, Galbrecht et al. (1959) presented information concerning SR, RR, HR. components of the OR in humans. The SR component was most consistent. The SR component clearly decreased in magnitude as a function of trials, yet failed to extinguish completely in a series of 18 tones spaced at 1-min. intervals. (Curah & Stern, 1963) reported adaptation of the SR component of the OR in children, who exhibited quicker habituation the second day then on the first. They also reported habituation of spontaneous activity in SR (non-stimulus coupled oscillations), which neither we (Wilson & Dykman (1963), Lacey and Lacey (1958) nor Johnson (1963) found.

Figure 2 shows for the left side only the mean scale score in skin re-sistance for each tone in each of the four sessions.

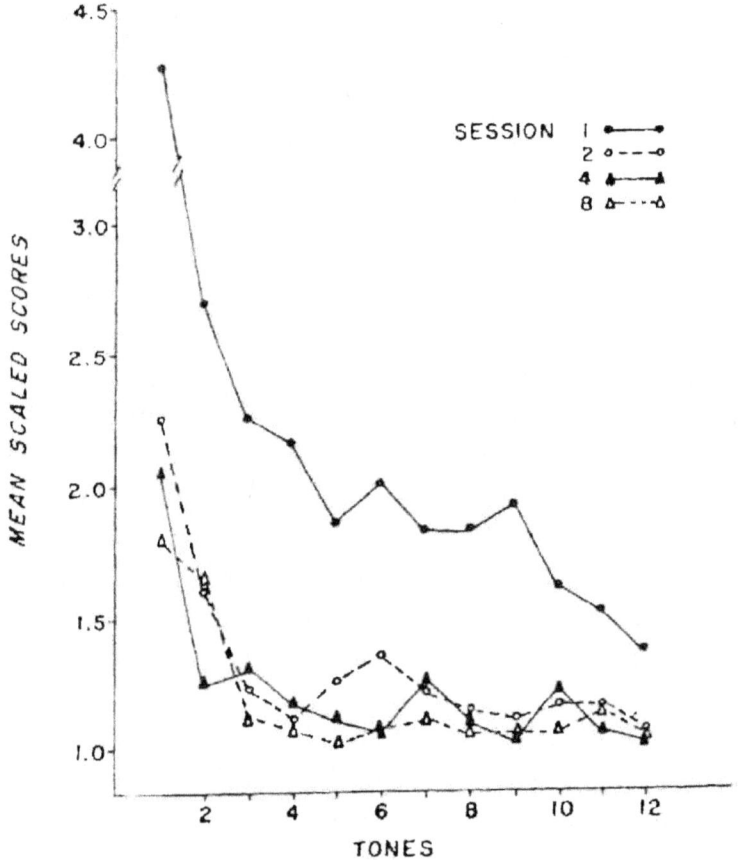

Figure 2 Mean scale scored in SR (left side) for each tone in each of four sessions.

Figure 3 shows the mean difference in skin resistance for each tone in each of the four sessions. Again we show only the left side because the right side was almost identical to the left side.

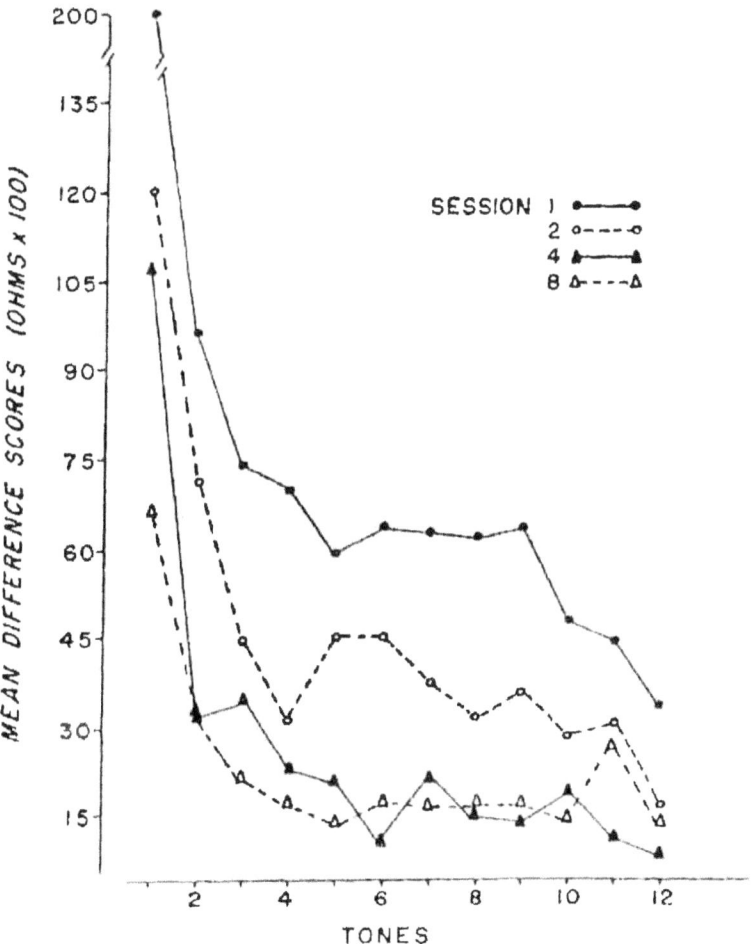

Figure 3 Mean difference score in SR (left side) for each tone in each of four sessions.

Table 1 shows the coefficients of concordance (agreement) across daily sessions for heartrate, repertory rate, skin resistance (left), and muscle potentials (left). We did not show the figures for the right because the figures on the left were very similar to those on the right. N=40 junior medical students.

TABLE 1

COEFFICIENTS OF CONCORDANCE ACROSS DAILY SESSIONS *

System	Stimulus Levels	Scaled Scores	Diff. Scores	S/PS Ratios
HR	.62	.47	.48	.52
RR	.70	.59	.51	.52
SR (left)	.67	.33	.44	.42
MP (left)	.53	—	.38	.33

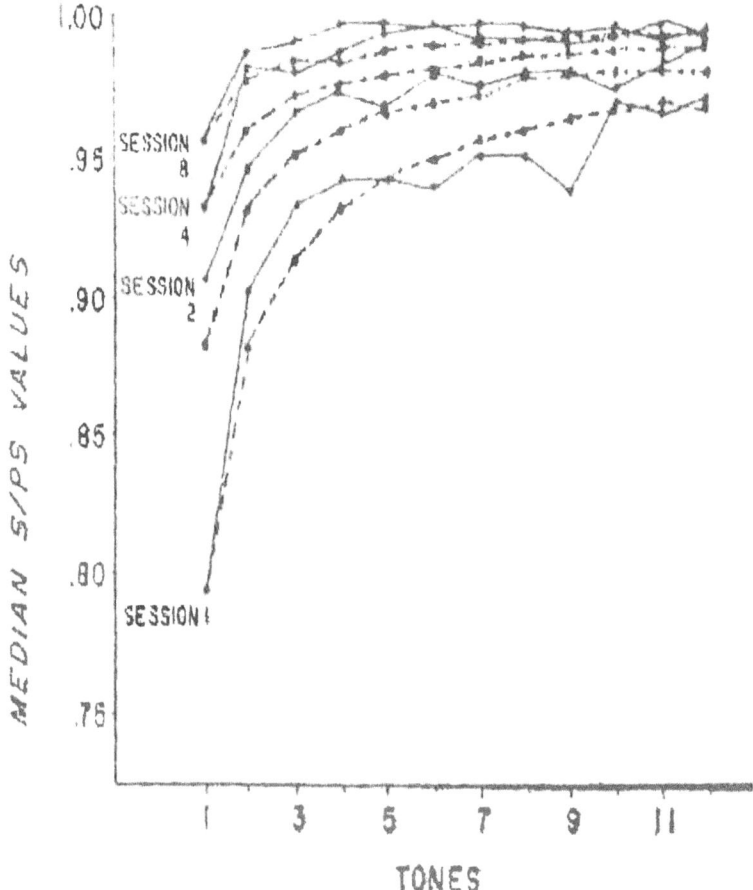

Figure 4 Median S/PS values in SR (left side) for each tone in each of four sessions.

Figure 4 is important because it shows the effect of partial extinction as a function of the number of trials. It never completely disappears.
The formula for figure 4 is shown below.

$$(S/PS)^t = 1 - \left[\left(D^{(0.8)} \right) \left(T^{(0.8)} \right)^{\overline{k}} \right]$$

The formula above $(S/PS)^t$ is the predict value of the median on any trial and day. D is the session number (1-8), and T is the trial number (1-12). K is a constant equal to $1-(S/PS)^t$. S_1 is the stimulus level, and PS is the prestimulus level for the first tone on the first day. A number of mathematical equations were applied to the empirical data, but the hyperbolic function appeared by inspection to provide best fit. This formula shows the median S/PS values in SR (left side).

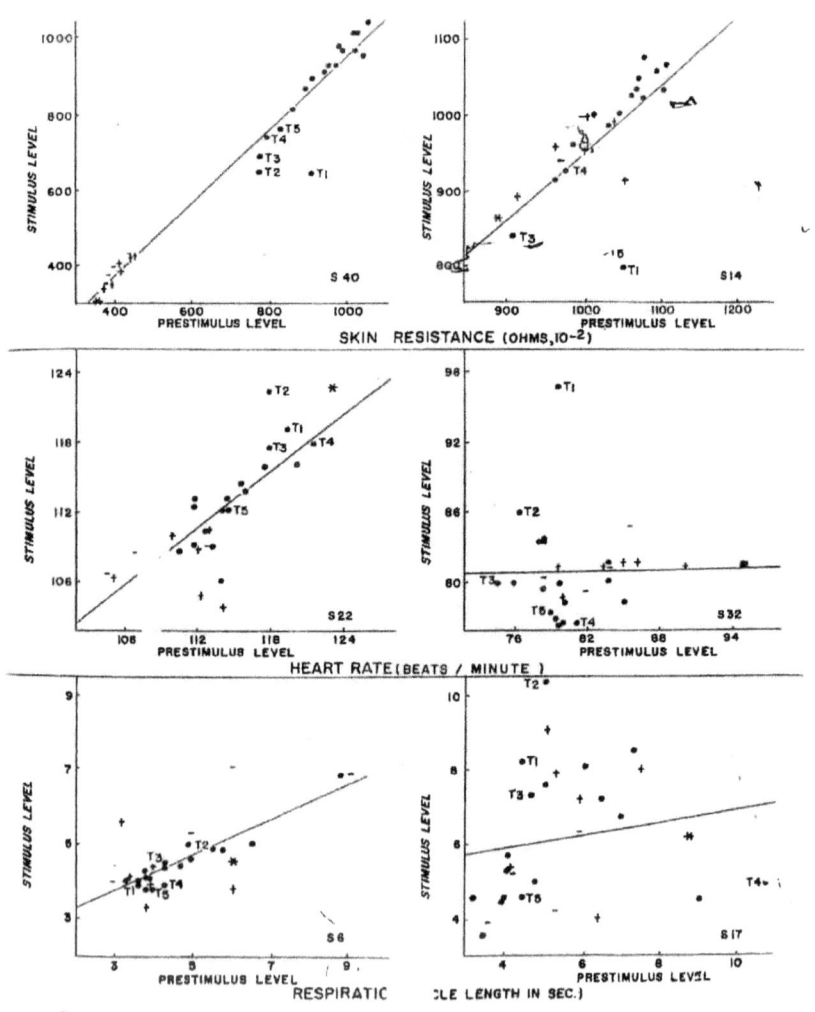

The experiment began almost immediately following the placement of the electrodes. It consisted of three phases: a rest, tone, and question period. Basal recordings were made for 5-min, followed by a series of 12 tones, each 800 Hz, 60 dB, and 5-sec. in duration. The intervals between tones were 1 min. ± 5 sec. This enabled the program we wrote for recording equipment to present tones at the peak of inspiration. Following the tones participants heard a series of 11 questions. Odd numbered questions except for the last were neutral in emotional content except for the 11th. The even numbered questions were designed to initiate an emotional response. The questions were short (e.g., How many seconds in a minute? How do you feel about your studies?) Subjects were instructed to think of questions without answering them out loud. Questions were given at the rate of one per minute. The experiment ended with a stimulus free period 3 minutes long. It was not possible or necessarily even desirable, to run students on consecutive days. Inter-session intervals varied from 2 to 3 days, a better test of extinction than a test every day.

The top figure on the left (Figure 6) shows the results just for skin resistance and it can be seen that the prestimulus levels and the stimulus levels are correlated. However, when you look at the graph you notice that the tones which appeared first in time are well below the best fitting line (tone 1, 2, 3, 4, 5). These tones produce the biggest drop in SR. Of all the subjects, subject 40 had the biggest deviation from the best fitting line. The sooner you switch from low to high prestimulus levels, the response becomes less consistent. On the right side, the biggest deviations are T1 from the best fitting line. The biggest subject variation is subject 14 and has the biggest drop in SR. The graph on the right shows the results for much higher prestimulus levels. Here you can see T1, T3, and T4 are below the regression line. It should be remembered that the tones occurred before the questions. It turns out that things that occur first in time, whether emotional or non-emotional, dominate. This indicates that SR is a different kind of response than heart rate and blood pressure. They are more closely regulated by homeostatic mechanisms which Gantt discussed as an example of schizokinesis. You can see the graphs above show heart rate and respiration. They are far more variable than the skin resistance at the top which suggests that skin conductance is a different kind of measure than heart rate and respiration.

Figure 7 shows the mean T scores for the 40 subjects for each of the first 10 tones in SR, HR, and RR. T scores represent scores scaled in terms of standard deviations from the mean of all the scores. You can see the drop in SR is much larger in these scaled scores than it is in heart respiration.

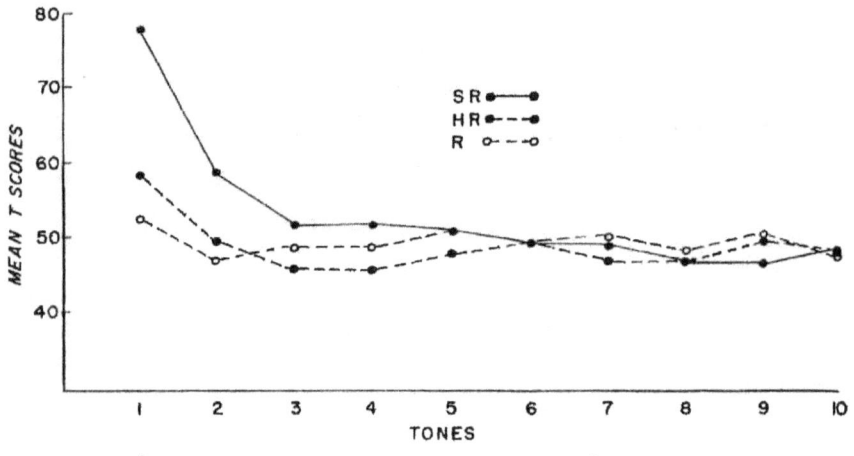

Figure 7 Mean T scores for the 40 subjects for each of the first 10 tones in skin resistance (SR), hear rate (HR), and respiration (R).

Propantheline Study
Juniper et al (1964)

PARTICIPANTS
Twenty freshmen medical students between 20 and 22 years of age were recruited as participants.

They received no information concerning the nature of the experiment other than that the study involved eight daily citations, and that they would be paid $20 per/ session. Each student was told that it was important to refrain from discussing the procedures with each other after they had been administered tests in the laboratory.

APPARATUS

The instrumentation is described in detail elsewhere (Dykman et al. 1959). In brief, SR was recorded by two Fels dermohmmeters, and two Esterline–Angus recorders, HR by a Fels cardio tachometer, and an Epsco galvanometer, RR by Statham strain gauge, Epsco carrier preamplifier, and Epsco galvannomitor MPs by Epsco integrator preamplifiers, and galvanometers. The Epsco preamplifiers and galvanometers were used to score the peak of MPs occurring in each 3-sec interval of stimulus-free periods. Knowing that instrumentation errors might produce systematic differences in SR levels on the two sides of the body, they were controlled by a random alternation of the two SR recorders during stimulus-free periods.

PROCEDURE

Students were seated in an upholstered chair with their feet resting on an ottoman. They were seated so that they looked toward the front of the room (opposite from our one-way viewing window), and were instructed to stay awake, and listen to the tones. The observation room was air-conditioned, and electrostatically and sound shielded. Two SR leads were placed on the inner surface of the plantar arch at the bottom of each foot. (Cup – type with zinc plat filled with zinc sulfate). Standard HR electrodes saturated with Sanborn jelly were attached on the left wrist and the right leg, depending on which recorded the larger HR waves. Respiratory rate (RR) was recorded pneumograph tube placed around the chest or abdomen at the point of maximum expansion. Muscle potentials (MPs) were recorded by EEG electrodes on each arm, placed 2 in. apart over the midpoint of the carpi digitorum sublime's muscles. A set of earphones, cushioned by sponge rubber, were placed over the ears, and students were left alone in the room.

Physiological Measures

Prestimulus levels of functioning were measured as follows: for SR, the exact level in ohms at the onset of each tone, for HR, the shortest interval between any two consecutive beats during the 5-sec. period preceding each tone, and for respiration (RR), the mean duration of the cycles just preceding each tone, and for MPs, the maximal microvolt reading occurring in a 5-sec.in any stimulus- free period. Stimulus levels for SR was the lowest level in ohms during a 20 sec. period following the onset of a tone, for HR, the shortest interval between any two beats, for RR, the main duration of the two cycles following the onset of a tone; and for MPs, the amplitude of the highest tracing doing each tone. RR was easiest to score, since tones were given at the peak of inspiration.

Results

We summarize the inter-session adaptation and extinction results for SR, HR, RR, and MPs. Important measures will be described below. SR provided the most reliable data concerning both adaptation and extinction.

Adaptation and Extinction

For convenience in exposition, we defined adaptation as a response decrement within single sessions, and extinction as a response decrement over daily sessions. On this point it may be worthwhile to point out that all terms commonly used to refer to response diminutions, adaptation, habituation, and extinction, are inadequate in one way or another. Adaptation generally denotes complex adjustments, habituation has as its root in habit, and extinction conveys the meaning of the complete disappearance of a response which is rarely (if ever) the case.

The pattern was similar for sessions 2, 4, and 8 (left side curves). But those for the right side were virtually identical. The extinction was clearly revealed across days – the SR drop in resistance to the first tone each of these next three sessions was lower in ohms then in the previous session. Adaptation and extinction were independent processes. Sensors were not codependence, and had to be measured separately. In a subsequent closely related paper, we studied palmar skin resistance and sweat gland counts in drug and non-drug states (Juniper, Blandon and Dykman, 1967). Darrow (1927) could find no constant relation between galvanic skin resistance changes (called GSR changes at that time) and local changes in circulation. He concluded that these two functions were largely independent. Darrow later found that the change in the electrical resistance occurred before the actual appearance on the skin surface suggesting that the changes in GSR occurred before the actual appearance of sweat on the skin. This suggested that GSR changes depend more upon electrical alterations in the sweat glands then upon the actual secretion of sweat (Darrow 1934, 1936). Woodworth and Schlosberg (1954), summarize research on the determinants of skin conductance, concluding that adaptation, depolarization, and permeability of the membranes of the sweat glands could account for resistance changes (p. 142).

Darrow came back in 1964, stating that the "recorded sweat activity is practically, if not entirely, absent during GSR responses." (We prefer the terms skin resistance (SR) and (SC) – the latter a reciprocal of SR). Darrow said, "Only when resistance falls to a certain critical level, here about 45,000 ohms, does sweating a company the GSR" (Darrow, 1964). Delbert and Wright (1966, p. 39) presented evidence suggesting, "That the palmer GSR involves the sweat glands, and an epidermal component, each responding preferentially according to the demands of the behavioral situation". They studied reactions to simple tones and lights used as alerting signals or executing signals in a perceptual were mortar reaction time task. For the reaction time task, the alerting signal was more potent in augmenting sweat gland activity than the execution signal. The opposite was true for the recognition task.

Background Activity

Wilson and Dykman (1960) studied the small fluctuations in SR that occur during stimulus free periods. Lacey and Lacey (1952) studied these in HR and SR. We used the term background activity (BA) to indicate atypical fluctuations, and background intervals (BI) to indicate time interval with background activity. Lacey found that errors in a stimulus discrimination paradigm gener-ated errors in a visual motor task. The present study differed from the Lacey and Lacey study by adding an addition al system respiratory rate. Participants were 40 junior medical students ranging in age from 21 to 32.

Forty junior medical students, all males, ranging in age from 21 to 32. They were selected to ensure heterogeneity with respect to scores on the Medical College Admissions Test (MCAT), and the Taylor Manifest Anxiety Scale (Taylor, 1953).

PROCEDURE

The subject were isolated in an electrostatically and sound-shielded chamber, with their legs resting on an ottoman. SR was recorded plantar arch of these, are, RR by a nomogram, and HR by conventional EKG leads the subject was observed through one – way vision mirror from the ad-joining experimental room.

The experiment consisted of three phases: a rest period, a question period, and tones. There were 18 tones, each 500 cps, (each 5 sec. in du-ration, and 40 dB above the noise level of the room). There were also open questions each given at 1 min, intervals. Participants were instructed to think about the questions but not the answer them out loud. Continuous autonomic recordings were made beginning with the last 8 min. of a 15 minute rest period, ending 3 minutes after the last question. Further de-tails may be found in the study previously cited (Dykman et al., 1959).

BASIC MEASURES

Each subject's record for each autonomic system was divided into intervals of 15 sec., eliminating the 15 sec. intervals which began with tones or ques-tions. There were in all 32 intervals during the rest. 54 during the tones, and 13, during the question period. Background activity in SR was scored as a decrease of at least 800 ohms within a 15 sec stimulus -free interval.

RESULTS

Most of the BI intervals had only one interval that could be scored as a BI. The percentage of BIs with two or more intervals of background activity was 8 for SR, 1 for HR, and 4 respirations. Table 2 shows the intersystem correlations of resting background activity (BIs) of three systems.

TABLE 2

INTERSYSTEM CORRELATIONS OF RESTING BIs

System	SR	HR	RR
HR	−.09	—	—
RR	−.09	.55*	—
MP	.57**	.48*	.35

* $p < .05$.
** $p < .01$.

Table 3 shows the number of BIs that could be scored in each system for the rest tone and question period.

TABLE 3

NUMBER OF BIs OF Ss IN EACH SYSTEM

Period	System	No. of Ss	p by χ^2
Rest	SR	16.0	
	HR	10.5	$> .05$
	R	5.5	
Tone	SR	21.5	
	HR	8.0	$< .01$
	R	2.5	
Question	SR	17.5	
	HR	11.0	$< .01$
	R	3.5	

Table 4 shows the internal consistency of BIs, the intersystem correlations of BIs.

TABLE 4

INTERNAL CONSISTENCY OF BIs WITHIN
EXPERIMENTAL CONDITIONS

System	Periods	r	Mean BIs[a]
SR	First 4 min. vs. last 4	.72	4.03/4.53
HR	min. of rest period	.66	3.93/4.21
R		.68	3.21/3.50
SR	Tones 1–6 vs. Tones 7–12	.49	4.91/5.11
HR		.67	3.47/3.39
R		.73	2.36/2.65
SR	Tones 7–12 vs. Tones	.70	5.11/4.80
HR	13–18	.46	3.39/3.81
R		.83	2.65/3.12
SR	Questions 1–5 vs. Ques-	.55	5.02/5.64
HR	tions 6–11	.70	4.86/4.34
R		.53	2.60/2.74

DISCUSSION

The research was stimulated by the paper of Lacey and Lacey (1958). We were able to confirm many of the findings although our experimental conditions and periods of scoring BI differed from those of the Lacey and Lacey.

Certain new findings emerged from our study as a result of including an additional autonomic measure (RR) and psychometric data. In agreement with the Lacey and Lacey, we found that (a) background activity is a relatively stable characteristic of humans. Participants maintained their group position in the number of BIs both within and across experimental conditions (b); and participants BIs in SR could not be predicted from his BIs in HR; (c) background activity is not directly coupled to stimuli (the time intervals closet to stimuli contained no more background activity than other intervals); and (d) the number of BIs of an S is unrelated to his levels of functioning (e.g., SR changes in ohms to specific stimuli). Although Lacey and Lacey did not study background activity in R, they found from inspecting their records that background activity was independent of changes in respiration RR. Stimulation (tones or questions) did not increase the number of BIs nor were there atypical oscillations in intervals close to stimuli than in intervals further away.

Method Study II

Participants

Propantheline Bromide Study: The group consisted of paid volunteers, two African-American women, three Caucasian women, and five Caucasian males. They were students, technicians, or secretaries 22-26 years of age. Table 5 and 6 shows the results for Propantheline subjects.

Procedure

Experiments began in the afternoon at least two hours after lunch. Participants sat in an upholstered chair in a relatively noisy, non-isolated room. They were permitted to talk with the experimenter, and watch television while the leads used in recording autonomic activity were attached. All experiments described for sweat glands were completed in the hospital (Juniper laboratory), where sweat gland counts were made, and not in our sound and electrostatically shielded rooms in the psychology laboratory, where more accurate measures of SR could be obtained with the equipment we had obtained from Fels (recommended by John Lacey).

Palmer SR, fingertip sweat gland count, and salivary flow were measured at 15 min. intervals, during a one hour basal period, and for 2-3 hr. period following the administration of the drug. The first five participants received 15 mg. of the drug intramuscularly. They had been told at the beginning of the preliminary basal period to expect an injection in about one hour. Because of the rapid onset of the drug affect after par central administration, the other four subjects were given 30 mg. orally. They had also been told when recruited that they would receive an injection of a drug.

Physiological Measures

Figure 8 is a photograph of the fingertip prepared for sweat gland count. The circled area is the area in which sweat gland counts were made. Fingertip sweat gland counts were measured by a modification of the Wada's technique, as employed by Juniper *et.al.* (1964). One finger, preferably the index finger, with a fingertip ring – pattern free of scars, was used to count the number of active sweat glands (see Figure 8). The fingertip was painted with a cotton swab that had been submerged in a 3% solution of iodine in 95% ethyl alcohol. When the iodine had dried, an access of a 1:1 starch–sterol paste was massaged into the skin with an applicator stick for 15 sec.

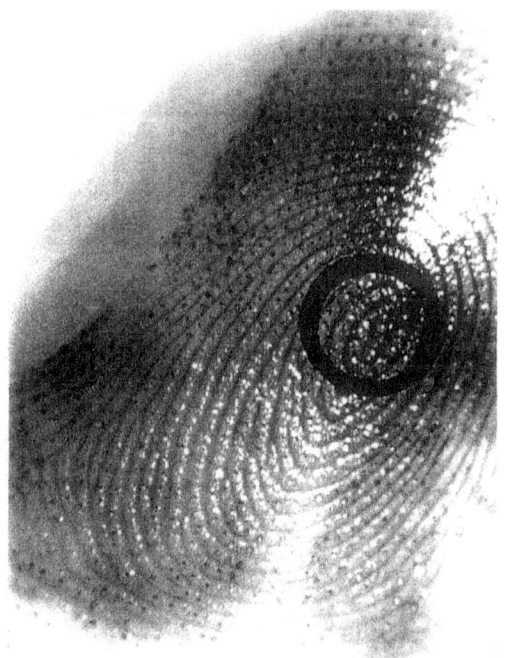

Figure 8 A photograph of the finger-tip prepared for a sweat-gland count. The circle indicates the usual area of the ridge pattern used for counting. Active sweat-glands produce black dots because of the starch-iodine reaction at the tips of the ducts.

Electrical SR was measured with the Fels Dermohmmeter, mentioned above, and standard zinc EKG electrodes supplied with the cardio–tachometer (Yellow Springs instrument Co., Yellow Springs, Ohio). SR electrodes were zinc disks 20 millimeters in diameter located in a plate holder. The electrodes were fitted with a jelly compound of 1%

zinc sulfate in 10% agar and 5% water. The active electrode was secured in the palm of the hand by a plastic clip. The reference electrode was strapped to the anterior surface of the arm with an elastic bandage.

Cropantheline Bromide Study. In seven of the 10 subjects, spontaneous and evoked SR changes of 10 to 20 thousand ohms occurred approximately every three min. during basal period. Propantheline eliminated these SR changes in all but one subject. This subject received the drug orally and exhibited little change in sweat gland counts. In those receiving the drug parent rally, SR changes disappeared within 3 min.

Figure 9 shows the reduction of SR in the Propantheline study. SR drops about 60,000 ohms (60 kilohms) as Juniper approached the subject with a hypodermic syringe. Following this large drop in SR, it climbed steadily back to about 90 kilohms. Note the smooth tracing in the post drug period, in contrast to the waxy basal control period tracing above. The drop in SR during the basal period reflects the anticipation of the injection. Participants told to expect the injection, showed a greater drop during the basal period than those told not to expect an injection.

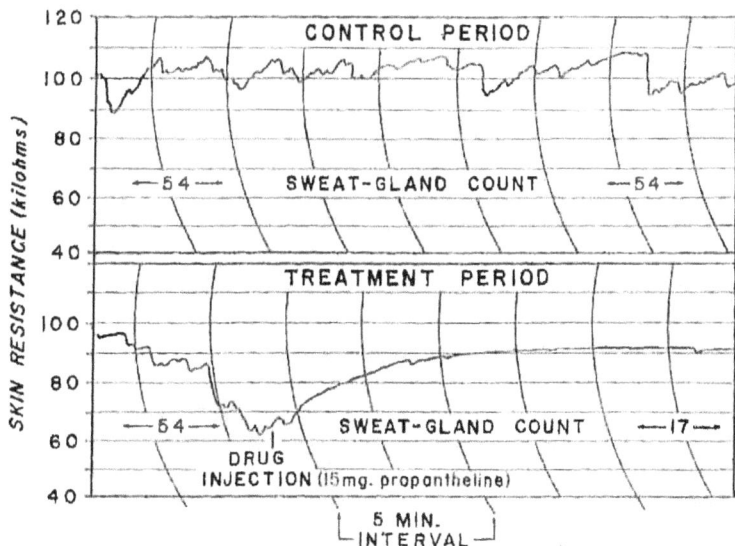

Figure 9 A reproduction of the skin resistance (SR) record of a subject receiving 15 mg of propantheline bromide intramuscularly. The chard was recorded from left to right.

Figure 10 shows SR values only at the time of sweat – gland counts in the basal period preceding the injection of the drug by 3 – 4 min. Had the SR record been read at the time of injection, the level would have undoubtedly been 10 – 20 kilos' lower than those shown for zero time in Figure 9.

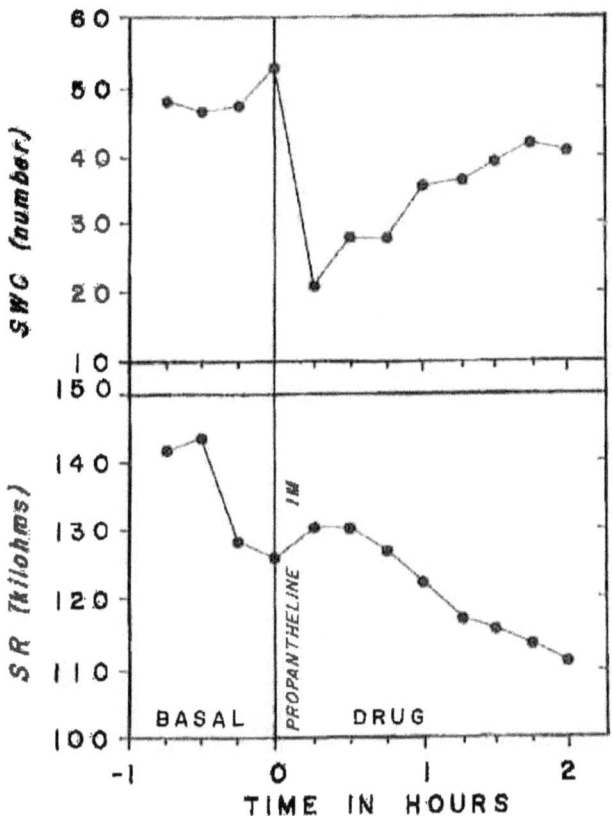

Figure 10 Mean curves of sweat-gland counts (SWC) and skin resistance (SR) during basal and drug-effect periods for 5 subjects receiving 15 mg of propantheline bromide intramuscularly.

Figure 11 shows the recordings we made of SR in the behavioral lab which are more accurate than those made in the Juniper laboratory. The small fluctuations in skin resistance at the top of the graph represent background activity. These are much smaller than the ones showed on the previous graph (Wilson & Dykman, 1960).

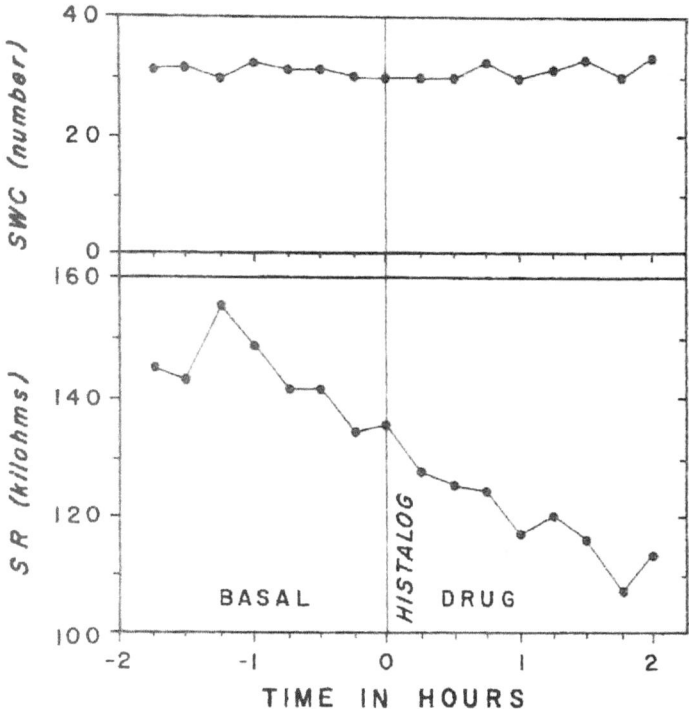

Figure 11 Mean curves of sweat-gland counts (SWC) and skin resistance (SR) during basal and drug-effect periods for 10 Caucasian males receiving 100 mg of Histalog subcutaneously.

Sweat gland activity decreased in the five participants injected with Propantheline. Following the injection, SR climbed for some 30 minutes and then decreased. The terminal decrease in SR occurred during the gradual recovery of the sweat glands. Figure 10 suggests that SR and sweat gland activity are independent. During the basal period, both sweat gland counts and SR were high, but this relationship reversed (low count with low SR) during the post drug period. The expected inverse relationship (hi count low SR) occurred only during the period of drug activity.

Figure 12 shows the Lisrel Analysis (Joreskog and Sorbom, 1993). This is a factor analysis of the Yale Inventory (Shaywitz, 1979). ACAP demotes Academic Aptitude, SATT Sustained Attention, HYP Hyperactivity, MYA MYTH Aggression, IMP Impulsivity, and SOC Socialization. The Mathews Youth Test for Heath (MYTH) has two components of Type A behavior, competitiveness and aggressiveness. We analyzed MYTH aggression, but the competitiveness scale didn't relate to any variables (factor loadings were near zero).

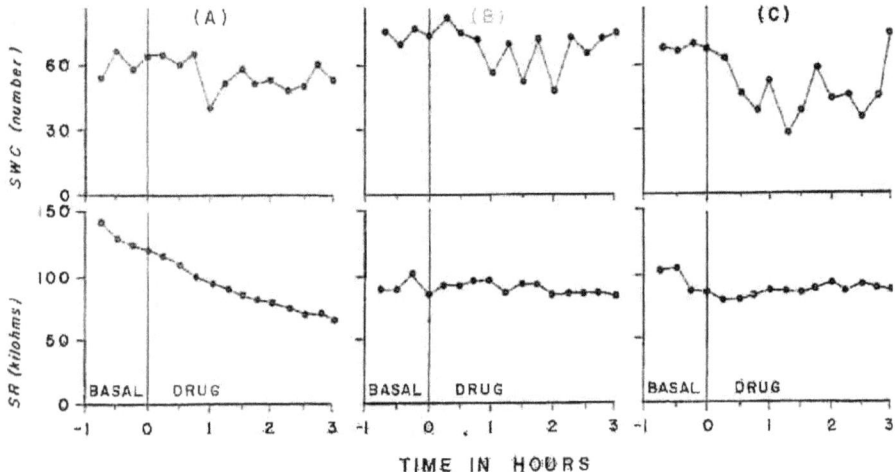

Figure 12 Curves of sweat-gland counts (SWC) and skin resistance (SR) for 8 subjects (A, B, & C) receiving 100 mg of Histalog subcutaneously.

The arrows pointing to variables such as ADD, Attention Deficit Disorder, is a term we suggested as a descriptor for the older term Minimal Brain Dysfunction (Dykman, Ackermna, Clements, and Peters, 1971). Lines ending on dug dosage indicate significant relationships by t-test (p<.01). The Loney Iowa scale or ADD included two of the Conners' variables, ADD (Attention Deficit Disorder, and the IHY (Iowa Hyperactivity Scale). Loney was the first to suggest that ADHD, the Attention Deficit Hyperactivity Scale as defined by the DSM, 3rd Edition, should include a component of aggressiveness. Turning to the relation IAGG and ADD,

IAGG had positive relation with ADD at the .05 level, but ADD was not significant in its relationship to IAGG.

Figure 12 (a) shows the effect of the oral doses of Propantheline which delayed the onset as contrasted with the injected drug patterns in the post-drug period for 12 subjects, which were extremely variable. This is the normal thing that happens when Propantheline is injected. Figure 12 (b) shows what happens when the subjects are told they are not going to get an injection. You can see from the graph that there is no response to a stimulus but there is some enhancement of background activity. This background activity is even increased in figure 12 (c) where there was still no stimulus. Now had we shown the subjects a hypodermic syringe, there would have been a huge drop in skin resistance (40,000 to 50,000 ohms). Interestingly, had we presented a tone, we also would have gotten a huge drop in skin resistance. Whether the skin resistance decreased to the tone would be larger than the skin resistance response to the threat of the syringe, would depend on which one occurred first. When a stimulus is introduced the result depends on which one occurs first.

Table 5

Intra-individual product moment correlations during the propantheline-active period

Group	Age	Race/Sex	SR and Sweat Count	
Propantheline Injected	36	N/F	−0.44	(8)[a]
	22	C/M	−0.84***	(8)
	20	C/F	−0.53	(8)
	32	N/F	−0.90***	(8)
	24	C/M	−0.96***	(8)
Propantheline Oral	26	C/F	0.42	(12)
	24	C/M	0.33	(8)
	26	C/F	−0.27	(12)
	26	C/M	−0.12	(12)
	21	C/M	−0.05	(12)

[a] The number of paired entries, from which correlations were computed, are shown in brackets. C is Caucasian, and N is Negro.
*** $p \leq .01$.

Table 5 contains the intra–individual correlations between SR and sweat gland counts during the period of Propantheline affect.

Table 6

Product moment correlations of all paired values for all subjects during the basal period, propantheline-active period, and both periods combined

Period	Group	SR and Sweat Count	Number of Paired Measures
Basal	Injected	−0.74***	20
	Oral	−0.40*	20
	All subjects	−0.74***	40
Drug	Injected	−0.74***	40
	Oral	−0.53***	56
	All subjects	−0.74***	96
Basal and drug combined	Injected	−0.59***	60
	Oral	−0.46***	76
	All subjects	−0.67***	136

* $p \leq .10$
*** $p \leq .01$

Table 6 shows the difference in basal drug and basal drug periods combined for injected, oral, and all subjects.

The next figures have nothing to do with the Juniper paper. Figure 13 shows the data from parents. It has the same Loney and Conners' variables as Figure 12. However, here the relation of IAGG to ADD was much higher than in Figure 12, a factor loading of .55. The reverse relation was zero. The parent ratings (parent ratings of hyperactivity in their children), ADD (Conners Scales), and the parent rating of internalization (introversion) and externalization (extroversion) Loney Iowa Scales had much higher ratings than those on Figure 12. The multiple correlation (measure of combined effect) as .92 explain over 90% of the variation in methylphenidate dosage. This is shown in Figure 13. When we reduced it to consider just he variables listed, the explained variance was 80%, which is very good. Figure 13 shows heartrate in high and low reward conditions and the different effects of methylphenidate on these two conditions. The low reward condition reduced heartrate much more than the high reward condition.

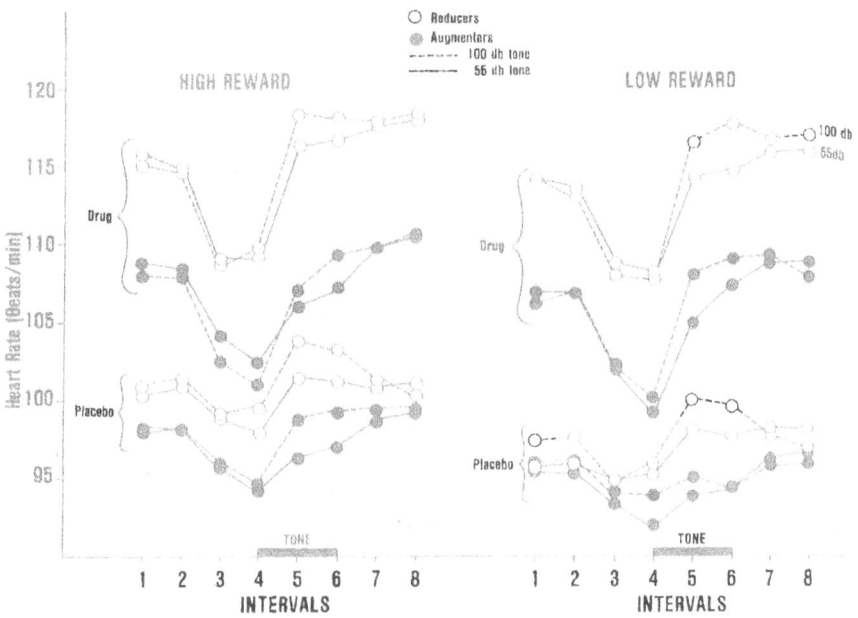

Figure 13 Mean heart rate response curves of augmenters and reducers to two tone intensities during high and low reward procedures and under placebo and drug conditions.

Figure 14 shows the factor analysis of the Yale ADHD scale; Academic Atitude, Sustained attention, Hyperactivity, Myth aggressive scale, Impulsivity, and Sociability (Shaywitz, 1979). You can see from these figures that the amount of variance not explained by Academic Aptitude is .30. The amount of variance not explained by Hyperactivity is .33. If you look at the two way connection from SATT to IHY, it is .13 but the connection from IHY to ADD is .45. Also the connection from IAG to IHY is .24, but virtually 0 going the other way. The amount of variance explained by IAGG is 33.9.

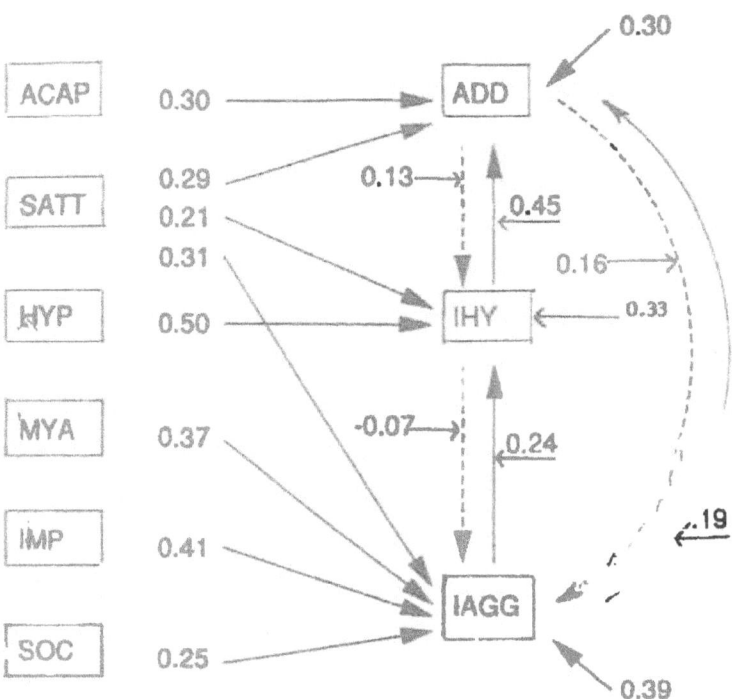

Figure 14 This figure shows only the statistically significant pathways (p < .05), except for 2-way connection. The significant 2-way pathways are shown by a dotted line.

Figure 15 shows the parent and teacher hyperactivity scale, the parent attention deficit scale, the parent externalization scale, and the parent internalization scale. The parent hyperactivity scale has a connection of .33 with ADD; .92 is not explained by that connection. Parent externalization (extroversion) and parent internalization (introversion). All the lines indicate the significant connections from one variable to another. Internalization (IAGG) fails to explain .81 of the variance. Yet its connection with ADD above explains .53 of the variance. The reverse connection explains none of the variance in IAGG. It's easy to read all these connections, so we will not spell them all out.

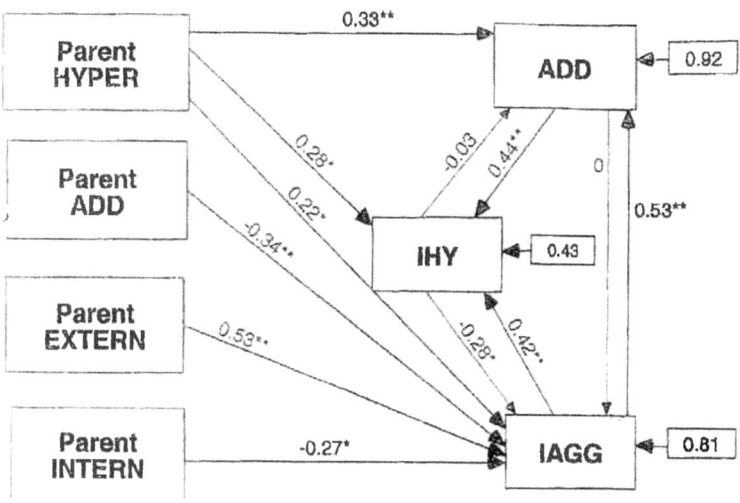

Figure 15

	ADD	IHY	IAGG	MYC	MYA	SATT	HYP	ACAP	SOC
ADD	—								
IHY	0.66	—							
IAGG	0.40	0.56	—						
MYC	−0.27	0.08	0.14	—					
MYA	0.25	0.57	0.68	0.41	—				
SATT	0.66	0.42	0.24	−0.36	0.01	—			
HYP	0.31	0.70	0.54	0.32	0.73	0.15	—		
ACAP	0.50	0.20	0.06	−0.34	0.02	0.38	0.13	—	
SOC	0.40	0.37	0.52	−0.29	0.35	0.28	0.25	0.30	—
IMP	0.27	0.45	0.69	0.22	0.67	0.05	0.50	0.12	0.34

Figure 16 It shows the correlations of all the physiological variables with each other.

Summary

It appeared to us that at first glance we had simply proven what Darrow had said many years previously (see Darrow above). The addition of Histalog, however, changes the interpretation. As expected, a 15 mg, of propanthe-line bromide, an anti-cholinergic drug, modified all skin resistance activity, except possibly those of less than 800 ohms which could not be detected with our sensitivity settings of the dermohmeter. On the other hand, following the injection of Histalog, sizable skin resistance responses continued to occur. Since Propantheline lowers sweat gland counts and Histalog does not, it would appear that skin resistance depends on some minimal sweat gland activity. This does not mean that SR changes will necessarily result in the appearance of sweat on the surface of the skin. The peripheral sweat – gland count is probably a very crude indicator of sweat – gland activity, although Wada (1950) states that a quantity of sweat as small as 0.95 micrograms coming from one sweat gland can be detected. It is certainly not sufficient to generate any measurable SR change; even with the kind of equipment, we had access to in our behavioral laboratory.

In the propantheline study, subjects told to expect an injection showed a greater increase in SR during the basal period than the group told not to expect an injection. It continued into the post – drug period. Whether the post–drug decline was due to Histalog, or to the normal discomfort of the gastric analysis procedure, is unanswerable. However, the collections of gastric contents were well tolerated by most subjects once the Levin tube was placed. In most experiments, SR levels gradually rise during periods of no stimulation. In studies of habituation of the OR, SR levels rise on the average, even doing periods of stimulation (Dykman, Reese, Galbrecht, & Thomasson, 1959), and (Dykman et al., 1963). Therefore, we still find tenable the hypothesis that increased basal mortar activity (Histalog affect) might "pump" more sweat into the skin and, therefore, lower the SR level.

Buettner and Odland (1957) found that the stratum corneum controls long – term diffusion of water across the skin. Normally, water flows outward but the flow may be inward if the relative humidity in the air to which the skin is exposed exceeds 86% (Buettner, 1956). Edelberg (1966) presented further evidence indicating a transient absorption from a moist environment and of the evolution of moisture into dry air. The inward diffusion is very rapid, and may occur when the sweat glands are producing sweat. According to Edelberg, "These findings are added to the evidence that the GSR is a two – component system consisting of a sweat - gland reflex, and an epidermal reflex, which may act together or separately" (Edelberg, 1966, p.93).

The low relations found between sweat – gland counts and SR in the present study seem to result from several factors. Counts and SR were not measured from identical loci, and the determination of active sweat glands is not as precise as the determination of SR. Two reports (Adams, 1966; Adams & Vaughn, 1965) provide excellent evidence that the sweat glands may be active without sweat filling the ducts. That is, the sweat gland secretions rise part way up in the ducts, fuses latterly into the stratum corneum, and are reabsorbed through the epidermis.

The stimulus level of SR is highly correlated with the prestimulus levels. Correlations as high as 90 or higher occur in very small samples; 20 to 30 cases is often sufficient, (Dykman et al., 1959). We did not find during serial stimulation, a progressive increase in the magnitude of SR responses, when prestimulus levels climb. It would appear that few stimuli (perhaps none, no matter how threatening) evoke SR changes as large as those from a relatively innocuous, yet unexpected stimulus (pure tones of moderate intensity) coming after a period of non-stimulation. Emotional stimuli of moderate intensity elicit SR changes just as large as more traumatic stimuli, provided the moderate stimuli precede the more traumatic stimuli (Dykman *et al.*1963). If the magnitude of the SR response were strictly proportional to the significance of the stimulus, there should be no attenuation of response with trials. Therefore, mechanical factors beyond those underlying habituation are implicated – perhaps fatigue of the sweat glands, or increased efficiency of reabsorption mechanisms, or both. Whatever, the mechanisms, there are no parasympathetic constraints on SR that "set" the same precise limits on functioning, as is the case for HR. For most autonomic functions, these constraints ensure some untapped reserves to meet new emergencies (Dykman *et al*, 1963). The split of these functions is another good example of what Gantt (1946, 1953) referred to as schizokinesis.

We did a large number of studies of skin resistance (SR), heart rate (HR), blood pressure (BP), muscle action potentials (MPs), in which participants were children with a diagnosis of ADHD, or adult hospitalized patients. Most of our experiments began with the recording of basal or resting levels for 8 to 10 minutes. As stated above, (Darrow, 1929) found that when subjects turn attention out to process environmental stimuli, HR decreases. But in solving problems in mental arithmetic, attention turns in and HR accelerates as they shut out the outer environment. They might say "Do not bother me; I am trying to learn a math soliloquy". We recorded alpha activity from expert meditators. All of them were very good at sustaining alpha. One of the teachers of meditation was able to maintain alpha for an hour, something never seen this steady basic resting rhythm in an adult. Diner, Holcomb, & Dykman (1985) reported differences in the P300 component of the event related potential between major depressed patients and normal controls. Darrow (1927) found no consistent relation between the GSR (galvanic skin resistance response) and local changes in circulation. He concluded that the two functions are independent. In 1934, he discovered that skin resistance (SR) decreases long before the actual appearance of sweat on the skin, and in (1964) he reported that the sweat glands do not secrete fluid until skin resistance decreases by at least 15,000 ohms.

Savant Syndrome

This often coincides with the disorder such as autism, but may occur independently as a diagnosis. It is not recognized as a mental disorder in medical manuals in either ICD – 10 or in DSM – V. Almost all people who have this disorder have exceptional memory, but have some difficulty in putting it to use (Treffert, 2009). Many of these people are famous for their achievements in the music, engineering, art, sculpturing, painting, and in other fields. The most interesting Savants are those with calendar memories, which occurred in one pair of them is identical twins (George and Charles Finn), described by Oliver Sachs (1985). If you told either of the twins a date, say May 5, 1760, he could provide the day of the week this date occurred. Normal people can also learn to do this, by memorizing the steps in a relatively complicated mathematical coding system (see The Secrets of Mental Math, by Arthur Benjamin, 2011, pp, 148-164, published by The Great Courses). After you look at this chapter, you will be asking yourself, how in the world could the twins do this? There may have been books describing procedures for doing this that they read. The IQs for savant's ranges from severely retarded too exceptionally bright (perhaps a range of all possible scores). The Savant Syndrome occurs in some autistic children, and surprisingly, some of these, borderline in intelligence, have exceptional memories, so calendar memory is likely an independent ability, separate from those diverse mental abilities that define IQ.

Nancy Andreason On Creativity

Recognizing that the importance of types of humans; whether of body or mind, is a debatable issue. I was impressed with an article Nancy Andreasen wrote for Atlantic Monthly (July 2014) reviewing the work of Terman in the literature which describes the family history of geniuses such as Einstein and Newton. The participants in these reviews appear to be two different branches of the human tree. Of the some 1000 bright children in elementary school that Terman (1916, 1937, and 1960) recruited for his study using his Stanford Binet Intelligence Scales, none turned out to be geniuses even though they had IQs over 135. They did grow up to be healthier, more athletic, attractive, and socially mature than a comparison group. Andreasen noted that William Shockley, who was 12 years old in 1922, "When the students (called Termites recognizing Terman) somehow failed to make the cut for the study, even though it would go on to share a Nobel Prize for the invention of the transistor." (Andreason, 2014).

Does Iq Predict Outstanding Creativity? No!

The mean IQ score on the Stanford Binet is 100 with average scores ranging from 85 to 115, and about 156/1000 adults have IO scores above 115. Terman (1916) selected 1000 elementary and secondary school children with IQs of at least 135. The high IQ scores of those recruited for the study turned out to be an excellent predictor of school grades. This is no surprise considering most of the children came from good homes, containing many books and other educational materials. More important, they were born from bright parents who cared very much about the education of their children.

One might think that Terman should have found at least one adult genius in the 1000 children he followed into adulthood. An IQ of 135 occurs in about 9 adults/ 1000. Only 1/1000 has an IQ of 145 or higher. IQs of 156 occur about once in 100,000 tests (estimates rounded to the nearest whole number). True geniuses such as Einstein, Edison, Galton (Father of Behavioral Genetics) are extremely rare – perhaps one in a million or more. Therefore, from a statistical standpoint, it is extremely unlikely that Terman would have found one true genius in his sample of 1000 children. I had three very bright Chinese students that I helped to obtain MS degrees in signal processing, very high grades (all were A students in engineering), but no better than my American students in repairing and operating laboratory equipment.

Andreasen describes a number of people generally recognized as intellectually gifted, who committed suicide, or had mental problems of their own, including first and/or second-generation relatives with psychiatric problems. The evidence presented is sufficiently convincing to believe that there is a positive relationship between genius and the co-occurrence of pathological conditions such as depression and schizophrenia. Some research indicates that creativity is more likely to be found in with IQ scores closer to 110 to 135 or higher. Andreessen's brain imaging studies, particularly those for functional magnetic resonance imaging (fMRI) reveal differences in brain functioning between adults recognized for their highly creative achievements, far removed from Newton, and others of similar merit. Andreasen points out some amazing feats of memory for ordinary people. The following quote comes from her paper.

"For example, we know that London taxi drivers, who must memorize maps of the city to earn a hackney's license, have an enlarged hippocampus – a key memory area – as demonstrated in

magnetic resonance imaging… Imaging studies of symphony or-chestra musicians have found them to possess an unusually large role Broca's area – a part of the brain in the left hemisphere that is associated with language." (Andreason, 2014).

Dr. Nathaniel Kleitman (1895-1999)

His long life may be attributed in part to the fluid diet he went on for a month every year while a professor of physiology at the University of Chicago. He was my principal research advisor. In addition to his knowledge of physiology and conditioning, he was known as the Father of Sleep research. From him, I learned much more about physiology. I first met while auditing a medical school course in physiology. Before accepting me as a graduate student, he made me read the first edition of the classic book on conditioning published by Hilgard and Marquis (1940). He also recommended that I read the English translation of the research of Pavlov by G.V. Anrep (1960). This was a new revision of the original book, and includes all the material first published in 1927 by Oxford University Press, as well as changes in Pavlov's thinking to the time of his death (1936). From all the above sources, I learned much about Pavlov's personal life and his physiological theories of conditioning. These books just mentioned, and those of Gantt, whom I would later meet, are still available at Amazon.

Kleitman recommended that I begin my spinal conditioning research by studying animals lower on the phylogenetic scale then cats or dogs. He thought that spinal cord might be more important and the brain less important in regulating reflexes in these lower species. I began with frogs, because I could not find any dinosaurs, which supposedly had two brains, one front and one back, and found that frogs with transected spinal cords died in a few days. It occurred to me that they might need to be cooled, and I tested their survival by placing them in in the food compartment of a refrigerator set at 40°F. This extended the survival time of every frog, allowing more time for the test of conditioning. The frogs exhibited the crossed – extensor (walking) reflex, when either hind limb was stimulated with very low amperage current, first described by Sherrington (1906). Unfortunately, I could not find a CS that would elicit a CR when the UCS followed the CS (tones, pinpricks, bubbling water, etc.)

Kleitman and his graduate students did the classic early sleep research. This research was the foundation for everything, which came later, and is described by R.T. Pivik in the Handbook of Psychophysiology (edited by J.T. Cacioppo, LG. Tassinary, & G.G. Bernston, 2000). Pivik, a very good friend and collaborator, took over my job at Arkansas when I moved to the Neuropsychology Laboratory at the University of Louisville in 2004. He described the early history of sleep, in Ban and McGuigan (1987):

"Early theories attributed sleep to various changes in the distribution, temperature, or constitution of blood, and considered the difference between sleep and death simply a matter of degree" (Kleitman, 1963). Later concepts extending into the earliest 20th century localized sleep to the brain and described many functions to this state including enhancing digestion, creating new 'animal spirits' required for waking behavior, and eliminating potentially harmful 'humors' from the body (Wittern 1989). Paralleling these notions were beliefs that dreams contain messages foretelling the future, revealed tor illnesses, or provided unique access to the unconscious (Kramer, 1994; Webb, 1993).

The most important studies on the nature of sleep physiology, and psychology, can be traced to the mid-20th century, when a graduate student of. Kleitman, Eugene Aserinsky, observed episodes of rapid eye movements (REM) associated with dreaming (Aserinsky. 1996). This led to a series of studies that focused on the neurophysiological stages associated with sleep (Aserinsky & Kleitman, 1953, 1955, Dement 1955, Dement & Kleitman, 1957 a, b, including many studies by Dement detailing the electro-physiological stages of sleep."

Phil Shurrager (1993-2003)

Shurrager wrote the paper that was eventually published on my spinal conditioning research without contacting me (Dykman & Shurrager, 1956). The research was completed in 1949, and the first published mention of the spinal cord research was the walking behavior paper, published in 1951 by Shurrager & Dykman. Shurrager praised the ingenuity of the Russian investigator Franzisket (1951) for his invention of the refrigeration process. I resented this praise, because he ignored or had forgotten the research I had done on refrigeration when he first hired me in about 1946.

Dr. Kleitman suggested some additional operations on kittens to demonstrate that the spinal conditioning reported was a forward process, defendant upon CS before UCS and not the reverse. However, he did not know nor did I, at that time the pairing of the CS with the UCS is not as important as the linear relation between the CS and the UCS. Conditional and unconditional stimulate were randomly alternated, with a random variation of times of presentation of 2 to 5 seconds between stimuli, without ever being paired. This procedure did not present any evidence of either forward or backward conditioning. After doing this, I was not in the mood to operate on any more kittens.

Russian studies reported by Pavlov (1927-1928), summarized by his student Asratyan (1972) indicated that all conditioning was both a forward and backward process. In the same paper, Asratyan described in details his own ideas about dual processing, without neglecting the founder, Pavlov. Cautela (1987) wrote a chapter on backward conditioning in which he first described the work of Rescorla (1967).

"In 1967, Rescorla made a contribution to experimental methodology in investigating backward condition (62). He introduced a true random control procedure to eliminate the influence of non-associative factors and to reduce the possibility of transforming the excitatory experimental CS-US contingency into an inhibitory

contingency. In the Rescorla procedure, the conditional stimulus (CS) and the unconditional stimulus (US) are unpaired. They are both presented but never close in time. A specific example of Rescorla's random control is the pairing of a US with one CS but not another. Rescorla considers the backward conditioning procedures to be a prime example of forward inhibitory conditioning, since the occurrence of the CS predicts a period free of the US."

Now this experiment is no different whatsoever from what we did in studying autonomic conditioning (Dykman, Whitehorn, & Gantt, (1955). We did not find any difference in either the forward or backward conditioning procedures. We did not however take into account the experiments Gantt did on the timing of pairings of CS and UCS which will be described in detail below.

Cautela describes his research which followed that of Rescorla. The conclusions that Cautela arrived at, were as follows:

1. *The results of a number of experiments can be attributed to either pseudoconditioning or sensitization.*
2. *In some cases where an aversive stimulus is employed as the US, conditional inhibition has occurred. This inhibition is associative conditioning but due to a forward pairing where the CS acts as the signal for the nonoccurrence of the US.*
3. *In all but two experiments reporting genuine backward conditioning, aversive US have been employed.*
4. *Backward conditioning has been reported in two studies employing an appetitive US. In one study by Antonova employing food as a reinforcer, it is clear that the CS was presented contiguously with the eating of food (2). In another study, by Rudenko and Struchkov, the results can be attributed to forward conditioning as a result of secondary reinforcement of the fractional antedating goal reaction (65).*

5. *Some studies reporting backward conditioning had unstable and readily disappearing CR. These data are not isomorphic with the data on forward conditioning.*
6. *For the most part, theoretical models of backward conditioning preclude backward conditioning as a true conditioning phenomenon.*

…It is my position that backward conditioning cannot be considered genuine conditioning until two conditions are met: 1) the backward conditioning data must exhibit the same properties as forward conditioning without the use of an aversive stimulus; 2) simultaneous condition with an appetitive US must be ruled out.

He appears to be saying that the forward conditioning is so dominant the backward conditioning is almost virtually impossible.

Cautela (1987) wrote an article showing that most backward conditioning that has been reported is actually forward conditioning. Dykman, Gantt, & Whitehorn (1955) published a paper for Psychological Monographs on heart rate conditioning suggesting that both conditioning and differentiation were dependent upon emotional sensitization. Dykman (1976) theorized that the first physiological alteration in conditioning is sensitization. I now believe that all learning begins with emotional sensitization. As I looked into the matter of sensitization with the walking behavior paper published in 1951, I decided that I needed more time to think about the issue of sensitization before publishing the spinal conditioning paper. However, Shurrager "beat me to the punch," publishing without my knowledge, the first paper on my spinal conditioning research, in 1956, some seven years after the studies were completed. (Shurrager & Dykman, 1951).

I attended psychological meetings in New York and elsewhere where I described the spinal cord research. I have clippings of articles from the New York Times; one in 1949 with the heading, "Scientist discovers hind brain in the cat." The New York Times also published an article on the walking behavior of kittens (1951) in which Shurrager's name was listed first with my name second. I realized that he was taking too much credit for my discovery. Shurrager also did a spinal transection on a puppy, and somehow managed to have it published with beautiful pictures in Life magazine with no mention of my name.

Shurrager's wife Harriett, who later got a PhD in psychology, deserves much of the credit for the continuing development of the Department of Psychology IIT. I remember her as a very nice person with excellent literary skills. She eventually received a PhD degree in psychology, and in 1958, obtained a large grant to study the intelligence of blind adults. Phil helped her with the research, and the test was marketed with the name, Hepatic Intelligence for Adult Blind. I did not look up the status of this test, but know that it was used for many years, after the Shurrager's retired to Florida in 1972.

John M. Stalnaker (1903-1990)

This is another tale of events going bad with a successful conclusion. While I was working with Shurrager, The President of IIT hired Mr. Stalnaker, then the Director of Research at the Association of American Medical Colleges (AAMC) located then in downtown Chicago, to review the work of the psychology faculty, and recommend changes for future directions. Mr. Stalnaker had completed all coursework necessary to obtain a PhD degree at the University of Chicago, and for some unknown reason, decided that the completion of a doctoral dissertation was a waste of time. He graduated with an MS degree from the University of Chicago where he was Phi Beta Kappa. During World War II, he worked on the Army – Navy College Qualifying Test, and was the Dean of students at Stanford University from 1945 to 1949.

The teaching staff in psychology of 1946-1949 consisted of only three persons: David Boder, Willard Kerr, and Roscoe Dykman. Boder was an eminent psychologist who wrote a book about the persecution of the Jews in World War II, saying, *"These are not the worst stories that could be told,*

I could not Interview the dead." Willard Kerr, a social psychologist, and a good friend, was concerned that I didn't have any publications. He worked with me in devising a collaborative study, comparing the worry patterns of psychologists and homeless people living on the streets of Chicago, with business people (Dykman, Heimann, & Kerr, 1952). It was interesting that this study, requiring only a few days of interviewing, was described in many newspapers and magazines. We found that the worries of psychologists and homeless people were statistically more similar to each other, than either of these groups was to business persons. Psychologists were interviewed at a meeting of APA, the business people in the Stevens Hotel in Chicago, and the homeless, sitting next to them, on street gutters in the slum areas of Chicago. Each homeless person was given money to buy an alcoholic drink in a nearby bar (all participants were males).

Mr. Stalnaker liked the progress Shurrager was already making in the area of Industrial Psychology, and recommended this as the sole trajectory to be pursued in the years ahead. After I left IIT, mathematical and statistical papers began to appear, more like those expected in a good engineering school. Shurrager and his wife Harriett deserve much of the credit for the elevated position the Department of Psychology now enjoys within IIT, the local community, and elsewhere.

Now for the bad news! Stalnaker saw no need for physiological studies, and recommended that I go elsewhere. I had never been fired before. I called Stalnaker, and made an appointment to talk with him, somewhat surprised that he would meet with me. I did not believe that he would bother to meet with me, and wondered if he had forgotten that he fired me. On the day of the appointment, and after I introduced myself, I said,

> *"What do you know about me? After telling me that all he knew was the research I was doing on conditioning, and that I was an experimental psychologist. I said, so it seems to me that you know little about my education at the University of Chicago or my reputation as a teacher at IIT. Many students in school with me*

*at Chicago will graduate in some specialized area of psychology.
I can do the same thing, and have decided, in addition to spe-
cializing in the area of Human Development, I will continue with
basic research on attention, memory, and learning in children and
teenagers. I have taught all the introductory psychology courses
offered by IIT with the exception of those in social psychology."*

Stalnaker seemed interested in what I was saying. Now, for the much-
unexpected news! He offered me a part-time job working for him,
which I accepted. One job assigned to me was that of checking the
answers on a forthcoming version of the Medical School Admission
Test (MCAT) for accuracy. I did find a few errors. When I left Hopkins
four years later, Stalnaker offered me a job as an Assistant Director of
Studies. He and I published the first handbook on the admissions requirements of all medical schools in the U.S. More importantly, we sur-
veyed the medical practices of women physicians, who had graduated
from medical school in the years 1925-1940 (Dykman & Stalnaker, 1957).
The American Medical Association provided us with the addresses of
the women physicians. Our study was cited as one that helped more
women get into medical school. My first class at Arkansas in 1955 had
only two women students, in 1955, but by time, I finally retired in 2004
over half the class. In addition, the attitudes of male medical students
concerning psychology and psychiatry gradually changed in a positive
direction as an increasing number of women were admitted to medical
school.

It is true that history repeats itself. Mr. Stalnaker was offered a position of leadership at the Merit Scholarship Corporation, which was
just starting, and he accepted the job. George Packer Berry, the Dean
of the Harvard Medical School, offered me the job Mr. Stalnaker was
vacating as Director of Studies at AAMC. Unlike the job I was offered
at Hopkins, I would not have to betray somebody I liked, if I accepted
this new job. I told Dr. Berry that I needed more time to think about
it, and arranged to meet with him in 3 days. I turned his offer over

repeatedly for three days, knowing a job would pay higher salary than the one offered at Arkansas. However, after going back and forth for three days, I decided to go to Arkansas, and work with Dr. Reese (Bill), so I called him, and told him that I was looking forward to working with him again. Dr. Berry could not believe that I could reject the marvelous opportunity he had offered me. It was a fantastic opportunity, and an opening for all kinds of jobs like the one Mr. Stalnaker was taking with the Merit Scholarship Corporation. The rejection of this job opportunity became even more unbelievable to Dr. Berry when I told him that I was going to move to Arkansas with friends I had made at Hopkins. At that time, the work of AAMC was supervised by the medical school deans, and from time to time, they hired somebody like Dr. Berry to look into the day-to-day operations of the Association.

William Horsel Gantt (1892-1980)

This section describes the research of Dr. Gantt, and his friends both literary and scientific that influenced his life. He was the last American to work with Pavlov. This section also reviews the research Dr. Gantt did over a period of 40 years at The John's Hopkins Medical School. Prior to one of his visits, we asked Dr. Gantt if he would be willing to participate in a videotape interview at the University Arkansas Medical School (UAMS) in Little Rock, He replied saying, "It would be an honor to participate with those of you that worked with me when you were at Hopkins". The tapes were recorded in November 1972, and they give an autobiographical background, a summary of his scientific contributions, and his much modest assessment of these. They also include his reflections on Pavlov as well as scientific and literary friends. After the taping, we learned that Dr. Gant had been suffering from and an attack of tic douloureux, which plagued him intermittently during his last 10 years, but characteristically; he honored his prior commitment for the taping. We did very little editing of the tapes wanting them to reflect his everyday conversations.

The tapes were reproduced in the first chapter of a book edited by F. J. McGuigan & Thomas A. Ban (1987, some 15 years after they were made). Because of the age of the book, it may be difficult to find. It contains assessments by 32 scientists, impressed by his research which was referenced by many of them in their original publications. Dr. Gantt never saw the book; he died in 1980. We will repeat here much of the book since it is difficult to find the original publication.

Three of the interviewers were close friends: Dr. William G. Resse (Bill) who had already completed his residency in Psychiatry at Hopkins, Dr. John E. Peters (Pete) who had not at that time completed his residency in Psychiatry, and Roscoe A. Dykman (Ross) who was working as a NIH graduate student fellow in Gantt's Laboratory. Ross was the only one doing laboratory research under Gantt's watchful eyes.

Bill obtained background information on Gantt's family history and his early work experiences. Each of us wrote a summary statement at the end of the chapter. Bill said in his, "although much his junior in age and certainly in reputation, I was treated by Gantt as a colleague, and even benefactor for introducing him to the VA, and in supporting him against false accusations of disloyalty to his country during the McCarthy era. Pete described some of Gant's friends, and his personal relations with the Gant family. In his summary statement, Pete noted that, "Dr. Gantt looked like a fearsome Mephistopheles, but his manner was so forthright kind and unintimidating that I immediately liked him. I (Ross) asked him to describe much of his research and its practical applications.

I enjoyed my personal relations with Dr. Gantt very much, but never called him Horsley until a few years before his death in 1980. He had many prominent friends that he first met while working in Pavlov's laboratory in Russia. These included Ogden Nash, H.L. Mencken, John Dos Passos, and Scott Fitzgerald. In some ways, Dr. Gantt resembled the Gatsby in the Fitzgerald novel. Like him, Gantt also had a party every Saturday night attended by the research staff and prominent people in Baltimore, but far below the conspicuous consumption of the parties Fitzgerald describes for Mr. Gatsby. Most of the friends Gantt had first met in Russia were deceased. Two of his very best friends, Dos Passos and Hamilton Owens, editor of the *Baltimore Sun* were younger men still alive in 1950. These two friends played an important role in defending Dr. Gantt when he was listed as subversive by the McCarthy administration (described in more detail below).

Bill: In his typical humorous way introduced Dr. Gantt in the taping session saying "Since you're known for your veracity, what were the date and place of your birth? We want honest account of the date". In the account that follows, I omit most of the parentheses.

Gantt: You state in a rather ambivalent way that I am noted for my veracity, then that you want an honest account. I was born October 24, 1892 on a parcel of land that my family was granted by George II of England. My ancestors came to that particular part of Virginia on the James River about 30 miles from Charlottesville. Dr. William Cabell came over in 1725. Another ancestor came over in 1642. My Gant ancestor came to Maryland in 1650. I am supposed to be descended from the Indian Princess Pocahontas. I do not know where her ancestors came from.

I visited his farm several times while I was working at Hopkins. The house in which the slaves of the Gantt family lived was still there. Gantt seem to have a deep and honest love for 'black' people (African American not used in 1950). We often met in the lab to have lunch with Dr. Gantt. On a few days, we had visitors to the lab. Dos Passos was a frequent visitor. The standard lunch was just cheese and crackers with some very good tea.

Gantt hired a new Ph.D., Sandy Stone, who received his degree in a French university (I think it was in Paris, but I do not remember the school). Sandy was an exceedingly bright and verbal person of Jewish Faith, and he had only been with us about three months, when Gantt described a trip to New York. He said, "As I was walking down the street, I saw some 'Negroes' playing craps in the alley." He then, turned to Sandy, seeming to know he had crossed a deep River, and said, "Sandy, Negro is a term of endearment in the South." Sandy did not hesitate for a moment replying, "Negro may be a term of endearment in the South, but it is a term of contemptuous familiarity in the north." It was obvious that Gantt was hurt by this comment, and he excused himself from the table and went into his office. It is not a good idea to say indirectly to your boss, proud of his southern heritage, that he is a bigot. In his dealings with people of all races, Gantt was opposed too, and fought against social injustices both here and in Russia. One of the things, Gantt liked most about Pavlov, was his open criticism of the communist government, at the time he was working with him. I have always wondered how Pavlov managed to escape the sword, during the early part of his scientific life. His Nobel Prize may have been a major deterrent later on, but his damaging remarks were started long before he won the Nobel Prize. Someone prestigious in governmental circles must have recognized his value as a scientific ambassador, both at home and abroad.

Bill: To paraphrase will Rogers, your people meet my people or my people meet your people.

Gantt: I value the fact that I like you Bill; was born on a farm, and had the advantage of the rugged life that existed then in the South, because the South had lost everything. The people in the South were rather impoverished. My father died before I was three, my mother was a schoolteacher earning $35 a month, and she encouraged me to go into medicine, since my father, Dr. William Horsley was a physician. I was originally determined not to go into medicine, and considered other things, but eventually I was more drawn to medicine than other fields. I received my M.D. from the University of Virginia in 1920, where I was frustrated by the life of an intern. I welcomed the news that Herbert Hoover was recruiting physicians to do

relief work in Russia. I applied for this job, and was accepted. I went on to Russia June 10, 1922 intending to stay three
months, bit having met Pavlov during that time, I decided to
stay on and learn from him.

Bill: Did you get into Russia via England?

Gantt: Yes, I went to England. It was a great thrill to see all those things
from Mother Goose such as London Bridge and St. Ives-- to see
all those places, which you really did not feel existed.

Gantt: After England I went through Germany and then on to Moscow.
From Moscow, I went to Saratova, a center of famine on the
Volga River. Then, I was transferred to a city known as Petrograd,
where I met Pavlov. My interpreter, Olan worked with Pavlov
from 1903-1094, and spoke good English. She encouraged me
to visit Pavlov's laboratory, and she took me there in October 29,
1922. Pavlov showed me some of his experiments, and from the
clarity of his descriptions, I decided to start working with him.

The nature of Gantt's planning for the future is revealed in the following
quote.

"I did not have any definite plans ahead. Most of my life, I did not
have any definite plans ahead-kind of living from hand to mouth.
I do not think I have ever made plans for the next year ahead
in all my life. I remember when I went through medical scho-
olong (his word). I never knew where the money for the next year
was coming from. I taught school a couple of years and made
enough money to get through the first two years, and then I do
not remember how I thought I was going to get through the last
two years of medicine. Fortunately, I had a cousin who made a
good deal of money in the shoe business in Lynchburg, Virginia.
I needed to get through medicine, and he lent me the money
to continue my studies. He did not get through the fifth grade
of school and went to work for a shoe company, and became

a millionaire. He happened to come by to see me when I was teaching school in Greensboro, North Carolina, and asked me what money I needed to get through medicine and let me that money."

I shall never forget my first day at work in Baltimore. I reported for work at 7:30 a.m. I was dressed in a suit, a new tie, and new shoes, the latter to my regret not anticipating a walk that I would soon take with Dr. Gantt. I walked up six flights of stairs in the physiology building to Dr. Gantt's office. No one was there and I waited until the secretary came in. She said he would come in about 10 AM, and true to her estimate, he came running up the stairs a bit out of breath at ten. I found out later the reason for the 10 AM appearance, he walked to work every morning from his home, a distance some 3 miles, and back to is home each evening. Each morning, he finished his walk with his dog before coming to work.

He immediately took me in to the suite that contained his office, giving me some crackers and a cup of tea. He had learned about my research on spinal conditioning from two people on my doctoral committee, who recommended me for a position in his laboratory (Shurrager and Kleitman). The committee included two significant others: Dr. Robert Havighurst, Chairman of the interdisciplinary Human Development Committee at Chicago described above, and William Neff, well known for his work on auditory perception. I do not know whether Dr. Gantt had ever visited with Dr. Kleitman. He would have surely mentioned him to me had he done so. Those of us who worked with Dr. Gantt knew by name most of his friends. Dr. Gantt appreciated the nice letter he received from Dr. Kleitman, recommending me for an NIH fellowship in his laboratory.

Dr. Gantt also asked me what I thought about Shurrager without expressing his opinion, and I simply told him without going into details that he did not treat me fairly. Dr. Gantt did not say anything, and I assumed he had heard this before from others.

After the initial interview, Dr. Gantt invited me to have lunch with him at the Hamilton Street club. Of course, I accepted, thinking we would probably eat in the hospital cafeteria. However, Gantt said, "Follow me" as he quickly walked out the door and down the six flights of stairs and out onto the street. He continued his rapid pace to the club, which was in the center of Baltimore, about three miles away. My feet began to hurt as I tried to keep up with him, and by the time we arrived at the club my new shoes had begun their job on my heels. Gantt introduced me to the various people there, but I did not remember any except Hamilton Owens, the editor of the *Baltimore Sun* newspaper. I would learn later that he would play an important part in Gantt's life.

I knew that as soon as lunch was finished, that he would start walking back to the Hopkins, and he did just that. I never said a word to him about my discomfort, and by the time we got back to the hospital, I had blisters on both heels. I learned some valuable lessons in walking with Gantt; you should be in good physical condition, be prepared for a walk, and bring a comfortable pair of walking shoes. I had thought of him as an older man, but he became much younger after the walk. He was 58 years old in 1950.

In 1951, I was invited to the main campus of the Johns Hopkins University to discuss my research. I talked about my work on walking behavior and spinal conditioning. I was pleased with the questions the Hopkins psychologist asked, and they gave me a very nice reception. At that time, Clifford Morgan was the head of the Department of Psychology. He had written a book on Physiological Psychology that had been revised before I moved to Baltimore (1950). I had studied his book in a Physiological Psychology course that I took as a student at the University of Chicago in 1946. Morgan's publications made Physiological Psychology a popular course in psychology at most colleges and universities. It was the first good book on physiological psychology. I talked with a professor (unnamed) in the department after the meeting. He told me that for the age of the faculty, his department had the highest number of scientific publications of all psychology departments in the U.S. After we had talked for a while, he asked me why I had moved from Shurrager to Gantt. I told him that I wanted to work for someone respectable and honest. He said, "In moving from Shurrager to Gantt, you have jumped from the frying pan into the fire." I was completely stunned not knowing what to say, so I smiled and said nothing more.

It is true, that Gantt had closer relations with physiologists and other medical personnel than with psychologists. Psychologists had burned him many times, even some who had worked for him. He asked me many times, "Why is my research not known or respected by psychologists?" I told him that much of his research had been published in journals or books not read by psychologists, and in foreign languages- Russian, French, and German. I angered him a bit when I told him one day, "You pay less attention to psychologists then they do to you". Russian research and that of Gantt emphasized long-term observation on a few dogs or human participants, the antiphrasis of most psychological research. Gantt believed that the type of dog, excitable or calm was more important in the development of an experimental neurosis than the environment, in opposition to the viewpoints of both B. F. Skinner and Pavlov. Gantt's concept of autokinesis was based largely on studies of one neurotic dog (Nick) studied over a period of many years.

Dos Passos, Dr. Gantt's best friend, visited the Pavlovian laboratory very often. He was very much interested in all the research that was going on there, and after seeing the dog Nick and reviewing his history, suggested Autokinesis as a descriptive term: the self-generation of different pathological behaviors over time. Gantt had already invented the term Schizokinesis to explain differences in the variation in the speed of conditioning and differentiation in different organs systems (heart, muscles, kidney, etc.).

I attended a meeting of one of the Northeast Psychological Associations with Dr. Gantt in which Neal Miller was discussing some of his research on learning (1951). As Dr. Miller started to speak, he looked out on the audience and saw Dr. Gantt sitting there, and said, "Oh, Dr. Gantt, I am so happy to see you. I have always admired you." Dr. Gantt immediately stood up, and shockingly said, "If that is true, why have you not referenced my papers?" I was embarrassed, but never mentioned this to Dr. Gantt, who invariably questioned persons who said things he did not hear or understand, and particularly something that appeared to him to be false. He did this to everyone; no exceptions. He said to a site visitor from NIH (Razran) for the largest grant he ever submitted saying, "Why are you here? You have worked in the same area as me, for years without referencing any of my studies." This may have been the only proposal Gantt ever submitted. Surprisingly, it was funded! He reported in the taping sessions that the first NIH money he ever received came from the NIH grant that I received to work in his laboratory in 1950 (p. 23, in the McGuigan/Ban book where the content of the tapes begin).

Ross: I want change the subject so that you can describe in more detail your studies, and some of the people you collaborated with directly or indirectly.

Gantt: Well you are qualified to talk about this since you are one of my chief research collaborators beginning in 1950.

Ross: Yes, that was a long time ago. I probably did my most significant work when I was working with you. I have used the methods I learned in nearly all the research I have done since I left your laboratory. While I was working in your laboratory, I was sometimes frustrated that my only job was research. I remember you telling me how lucky I was to have no other responsibilities. This remark made more sense later in my career, when my multiple obligations consisted of teaching medical students, writing grants, serving on grant review committees for NIH, and chair of the medical school admissions and other committees.

Gantt: Perhaps one of the most important projects to come out of the laboratory was your study showing that the heart rate and blood pressure conditional responses were proportional to the unconditional stimulus intensity. The blood pressure work was particularly important. It was the first to show the effect of both excitatory and inhibitory conditional stimuli. Another

63

important point that came out of your research was the retention of the heart rate and blood pressure conditional responses over 13 – month with no further reinforcement.

Hopkins: Gantt Vs. Adolf Meyer

Gantt: "During the winter of 1929, after I had been away for about seven years, I got a letter from Adolf Meyer, head of the Phipps Psychiatric Clinic, at John Hopkins. I had attended one his courses at Hopkins." He said, "I've heard of your work from John Dewey and Alan Gregg, the head of the medical division of the Rockefeller Foundation." All of those people had come to Russia and met me while I was working in Pavlov's laboratory. I had made acquaintances with prominent figures throughout the world. They had been told that there was a single American working with Pavlov. Adolf Meyer wanted a person with very broad interest, and he liked a lot of window dressing in his clinic. He hired people from various disciplines, part of the time just to confront them and show them that they were 'on the wrong track.' When he wrote me he said, "I think we might combine our mutual urges to advantage." I did not know that this meant an appointment at the Phipps (Hopkins Psychiatric Clinic). I did not interpret it one way or another. I met Meyer again in Boston when I came to the U.S.in 1922 for the International Physiological Congress with Pavlov. I told him that I thought I had an appointment to go to the Mayo clinic with Rountree. Myers made it evident that he thought he had given me an appointment at the Phipps Clinic, since he had volunteered to build me a Pavlovian Laboratory. I did not talk to Rountree anymore about going to the Mayo Clinic. I accepted Myer's offer.

In deciding my salary he asked, "What salary do you want"? I said, "I don't know what it takes to live in an in America, and I don't know what you pay people in my position." He said, "We pay them between $3000 and $6000 a year." I said, "I think probably

$3000 will be enough for me", and we settled on that salary. I did not know then the system of universities: they get you as long as they can and keep you as low as they can. It was a long time before my salary was raised to $4000. I got married on $3500 in 1934 (pp, 20-211) to Mary Gould Richardson. I heard later from people other than Gantt, that she came from a very prominent Baltimore family. By the time I arrived in Baltimore, their relationship had deteriorated. She would sometimes come downstairs to join his Saturday night parties, and occasionally attempt to embarrass him in front of his guests. He essentially disregarded everything she said. You always knew when Gantt set you up for an argument or ignored you when he was irritated. Gantt told Pete, who was a close friend of his two children, that he did not want a divorce until his children completed their education.

Bill: Hopkins had the policy that when you wrote a paper, it had to be approved by the department chairman. What happened when you submitted your first paper?

Gantt: Most of my papers had nothing to do with psychiatry. Meyer became annoyed when I wrote a paper on sex. When he read it, his cheeks turn red and he challenged me.

Bill: Was it canine sex or other sex?

Gantt: All of it was canine rather unsophisticated. So when I wrote the material gathered on the experimental basis for neurotic behavior, he held it up even though it had little to do with sex, and I couldn't publish it until after he retired.

DR. GANTT REVEALED his attitude concerning Myers saying:

"I did not feel resentful about much. I felt that if you elected to work with a certain person who was the head the department, you accepted his judgment about institutional policies. If you did not want to accept Meyer's judgment, you went somewhere else. That is a European ide, and I think it makes sense. You get

an integration of purpose by this method. Hopkins inherited this method from Germany, since many of the senior people at Hopkins had studied in Germany."

Bill asked, "Were you ever nervous about being scooped?" Gantt said, "No you had great security there – low demand for publications and funding from grants." Nonetheless, Gantt had well over 300 publications by this time he first retired from Hopkins in 1958. He went to Perry Point, Maryland to work with Reese, but only part time.

I complained to Dr. Gantt about the hold on my paper, knowing that it had to be approved by Whitehorn, who had replaced Meyer as the head of the psychiatry department. I said to Gantt that my career depended on publications. Gantt looked at me saying, "If your paper is any good it will be as good a year from now as it is today." "You are doing some very good work on blood pressure. It is important that you do not let anything interfere with that study." About a month later, Whitehorn asked me to come to his office, saying that he wished to review a paper. I was frightened, because the residences in psychiatry had told me he was a 'holy terror'. To my surprise, he told me that he liked my research. He arranged for me to see him an hour each of the next three weeks. He suggested that I should change the title of the paper to emphasize emotional sensitization. The paper that was eventually published with the title, Conditioning as emotional sensitization and learning, Dykman, R. A., Gantt, W. H., & Whitehorn, J. C. (1956).

Gantt did not say anything when I first told him that Whitehorn had suggested the title change, but it was obvious that he did not like Whitehorn's request to be included as an author. Moreover, Whitehorn did not raise his salary, and was attempting to force him to retire. In commenting about his feeling about Whitehorn, Gantt said, "Yes, everything is not exactly right in the universities. It became very difficult to live on $3,500. I knew that certain people who had graduated, and who worked under me, were paid considerably more than me. The financial people at Hopkins knew that these people would leave if they were not paid more.

Now, I would not say that I was not resentful of that sort of thing, but it did not bother me enough to try to go somewhere else."

BILL: YOU RETIRED temporarily from Hopkins at the age of 55, is that right?

Gantt: Well yes. I had worked with you at Perry Point, Maryland as a consultant beginning in 1950. Casey (Jesse F. – Head of VA at that time), knew about my work with you in the Perry Point laboratory. From him, I found out about the possibility of going to Perry Point. Although Dean Turner had been goading Whitehorn about keeping me on at Hopkins, Whitehorn had not come through with anything definite. Casey offered to build a laboratory at Perry point or Little Rock with you. I felt that this was a very big move to pull up roots and leave Hopkins, but I made the choice of moving down to Perry point full-time in 1958 at the age of 66. Turner invited me to continue to direct the Pavlovian laboratory in Baltimore, which I did on the limited part-time basis.

Gantt: An interesting thing happened when some people came over from NIH, and said they were considering supporting the Pavlovian laboratory. However, they qualified the offer saying, you should change the name from Pavlovian to something else. Of course, at that time, during the McCarthy era, there was great prejudice against anything Russian. They indicated that they could not fund the laboratory unless the name was changed. I always respected Turner for coming out and saying, "We like that name and that's the name it will always be."

This may have been a mistake, since they were going to provide money to support Gantt's laboratory, and it might have enabled Gantt to avoid the bullet Whitehorn offered of terminating his employment. I also knew that many members of the society at that time desired to change the name of the society.

The Pavlovian Society And Journal

Gantt: Howard Liddell was one of the persons who had been working in Pavlovian conditioning as long as I had or even longer (Liddell was a respected full-professor at Cornell). He wanted to form a group of people to meet and discuss conditional reflexes. There was no Society of this type in this country, and we wanted some kind of forum to discuss what we were doing, so we got together to discuss the formation of a group. Our first thought was that we would meet sequentially at Cornell, Baltimore, and Little Rock. There were just a few people at that time doing our kind of conditioning. Then later, I had the idea of making it interdisciplinary to include people from several domains of interest. I thought it important to keep some kind of balance in the society, and keep it to small numbers. I was looking for some 125 to 150 members from internal medicine, cardiology, and physiology, psychology with some people from other disciplines. I also had the idea that a healthy society should have younger people active in doing the work, and have mature people, not necessarily active experimentalists. Therefore, this was my conception of the Pavlovian Society. Then, after a great deal of mulling it over and advice from others, I got the journal started named "Conditional Reflex". The publishers wanted that name, but there was some division among the people in the society as to whether this was the best name. The Journal went all over the world even to a library in Peking. We had many articles coming out that had nothing to do with conditioning.

Ross: I remember Gantt running the organization with a relatively tight hand. Although all the officers had to be approved by the board of the society, I do not remember any that Gantt recommended being turned down by the board or the membership in a later vote.

THE BOARD CONSISTED mainly of past presidents. Bill Reese wrote the constitution for the organization with the help of Gantt. B.F. Skinner was invited to join the organization by Gantt, and he became one of the presidents of the society. Occasionally, I would join him in his early morning walk, when he attended the annual Pavlovian meetings. This was a great experience for me. Each president was elected for a term of one year.

It was in fact much easier to get articles published in 'Conditional Reflex' than in psychology journals. Over the years, and after Gantt died, the pressure to change the name of the journal, increased, influenced by an increase in members who were psychologists. Members with a medical school resume gradually disappeared. I hung on for years, and finally voted with the new members, for the name change, knowing that Gantt would turn over in his grave. The final name was Integrative Physiological and Behavioral Science. For a number of years, the society sponsored its annual meeting at the APA convention.

It became increasingly more difficult to get articles published, because the people that were appointed as editors instituted publication requirements similar to those for APA and APS journals. This supposed improvement decreased the diversity of the society, and people with a medical resume gradually withdrew the membership. Those still in research turned to other journals (many new ones), specific to their interests. The Pavlovian Journal was terminated in 2012, because a company willing to publish the Journal could not be found. Not surprisingly, the Journal was more popular in Russia than here, before the title was changed,

I suppressed when I voted with the members to change the name a good deal of the history of conditioning; for example, those wonderful experiments by Pavlov in which one UCS was made a CS for another UCS, turning an innate reflex into a conditional stimulus for another innate reflex. Hence, pairing works in strange and magical ways,

Joseph Vincent Brady (1900-1999)

Brady was appointed as the director of the Pavlovian laboratory in 1955, and worked at Hopkins until 1979. Before coming to Hopkins, he had trained three monkeys (Abe, Baker, and Ham) to withstand the stress of space travel. He was also noted for his work on baboons and his executive monkey study, including the establishment of a very successful behavioral therapy clinic at Hopkins. He was 89 years old when he passed away. I had the pleasure of traveling with him and his woman friend a pharmacologist, when the Pavlovian society met in Russia about 1982. When Brady replaced Gantt as the head of the Pavlovian laboratory, he wrote Gantt a letter saying, "I want to make it abundantly clear that your presence has always been welcome and appreciated." Gantt wrote Brady many notes suggesting changes in research and operating policies. Gantt was very happy with Brady's appointment and they became good friends. He encouraged Brady to join the Pavlovian society. Brady joined and quickly assumed a leadership role in helping Dr. Gantt manage the affairs of the society.

Dos Pasos (1896-1970)

Pete: Horsley, I think we can pass on from Pavlov and talk some about your own unusual life with people- the interesting group of friends over the years. The person that comes to mind first is John Dos Passos.

Gantt: Just a few words by way of preamble. It is interesting to know how certain rumors can get going about a person that are in so fantastic. I remember a fellow that came up to Perry Point and wrote a long article about me for Esquire, saying that I swam the Chesapeake two times in one week.

Peters: And the truth of the matter was you only swam half of the way out and back.

Gantt: The truth of it is that I only go swimming a few minutes, sometimes once a week, all during the winter.

Ross: But you actually did swim in the Chesapeake when the water was like ice?

Gantt:	Well, I did go in for short periods, but many years later, some-body published a newspaper article saying that I swam across the Chesapeake.

Gantt:	I met Dos Passos in Russia in 1927. There were very few people coming to Russia, and I met practically everybody who did come, because it was so rare. Most people who came had a letter of in-troduction to me or they knew about me, and this is how I met Dos Passos and Henderson. I was one of three Americans in Petrograd. The other two were people who were about my age now and had been there from early life. One was an old millionaire and the other was a schoolteacher in the royal family, and he had been around before the revolution. I met Dos Passos accidentally. He was at that time very much interested in the Soviet experiment as the "brave new world", and came to see what it was like. I met him up at a hotel where we had a good meal. He wanted to go down to the Caucasus Mountains. I had been there before. Therefore, we de-cided to go together and walk across the mountains. At that time, there was practically no official transportation, and you had to rent mules or horses or carts or whatever to go the 250 miles from the northern to the southern part of the mountains.

Although I never agreed with the political opinions of Dos, I remember discussing Bolshevism and what was going on in Russia, and trying to tell him some of the dreadful things that were happening. He still was not convinced it was not the best of all the possible worlds. He had to learn that for him-self. We took this walk across the Caucasus Mountains, sleep-ing on floors, and getting practically nothing to eat for about a week. The people themselves had hardly anything to eat. We heard that when we crossed from one military road to another that this place Zaramag would be flowing with good things to eat. This did not turn out to be true and then we stopped at a place where they killed a sheep. I remember being very sleepy waiting for the sheep to be cooked at 1 AM in the morning; the sheep was so tough you could hardly chew the meat. The hospitality of these people was remarkable; they would not take any money for the sheep.

We did finally get to Zaramag, looking forward to the good food we would find there. However, when we finally arrived, we were met with a cold rain and drizzle. The altitude was about 10,000 feet. We finally did locate a store, and all they had was about three-quarters of a pound of hard candy and six eggs. We were so dismayed we went back and slept on the floor in a schoolhouse, and the schoolteacher furnished us with some tea-leaves, but she had no utensils to make the tea.

Pete: Did you buy the eggs?

Gantt: Oh, yes, we bought the eggs and the candy too. You can imagine how dismayed we were when we had expected a week to find some good food. So then, we continued for about another three days down to the southern coast, and the shops there had abundant quantities of oranges and tropical fruits. Dos and I were happy to see this trip end. When Dos Passos left Russia, he gave me his shoes and his extra suit. It was very difficult to buy anything of that nature in Russia, and this gift of clothes was a great help. When I came back to America in 1929, and in I went to see Dos on Cape Cod, and we became devoted friends until he died about two years ago.

Ross: He was a famous author when you met him in Russia?

Gantt: Yes, he was well known then. He had written Manhattan Transfer and Three Soldiers, and he was well known in Russia because of his liberal views. Otherwise, they would not have let him in.

Ross: He became progressively more conservative as he got older?

Gantt: Yes, he went to Spain to help Loyalists. One of his very close friends who taught Spanish at Hopkins also went there to help the Loyalists. His friend was Spanish, and he was executed by the communists, What Dos saw there turned him definitely against the communist regime. That was about 1936. He became disenchanted with them from that time on, and he became progressively more anticommunist until, at the end of his life. He was always on the extreme right, supporting people like William Buckley. He never supported the John Birchers – he never got that far, but he really got very much on that side.

Ross: When I think back on the days I spent in Baltimore, I remember those exciting times we had over in your house. It was always a surprise to go there to see what new person you could meet. I certainly look back on it as one of the most fascinating times in my life.

Pete: I do too. This was a critical periods of my life that influenced me forever. It was always exciting to go over to your house and enjoy the tremendous hospitality that you and your family always expressed.

Gant: I think that was different from the way many Baltimore people think about entertaining. You do not have to entertain lavishly. You get the right people together and everything goes all rights. Dos Passos also entertained very simply. He had some good wine. Often, he did the cooking, and his dinners and entertainments were very simple. He did not like crowds, and was he very shy about talking. However, he was a superb listener. People would say to me after an evening, which Dos would have hardly said a word; "Oh what a charming conversationalist Mr. Dos Passos is; how interestingly he talks."

Pete: Did Dos talk much to you?

Gantt: We used to take walks together. Even after he had heart trouble, we took walks together. Ne discussed everything from relativity, gravitational fields to the speed of light, and Skinner. Dos was very much opposed to materialism. He was also against Skinner's idea of the external environment determining everything. He told me he enjoyed his conversations with Skinner very much, whom he met at meetings of the Pavlovian Society. He said that he was a very charming fellow.

Gantt's Loyalty Questioned

This section supplements what Gantt said about this issue in discussing it with Dos Passos above. It seems almost that much of what came up and his life involved his friendship with Dos in one way or another.

Pete: Did you and Dos discuss politics very much?

Gantt: Yes, we discussed politics and we discussed free will. He wrote in his autobiography called The Best Times about our trip across the Caucasus Mountains together. Dos Passos was a great friend, and he did not let political opinions or any opinions get in the way of friendship. He said he did not see why a person did not have a right to whatever opinions he wanted and why it could interfere with friendship. I think he illustrated the best qualities of a good friend.

Another example of his friendship was during the McCarthy regime when I was at VA at Perry Point. I was accused of being subversive. The flimsy grounds were "You're on the mailing list of the Maryland Free-State Bookshop. You were in such a meeting in New York and in this meeting you had an opportunity to meet communists. This meeting was a meeting of the Russian War Relief during 1943-1944. As you know, Ross, I kept a good deal of material that came to the lab. Therefore, I finally unearthed some material on this meeting, and saw that George Marshall, who was Chief of Staff, was one of the people at the meeting, and Vice President Wallace was present. Eisenhower was invited but was in Europe and the fighting had not ended. He sent a telegram saying he was sorry he could not attend, but he thought that every patriotic American should be there. So I wrote all this material down, and told Dos the night before when we were discussing McCarthy that he was doing a great deal of harm. Dos said, "No, he is doing a good thing getting all these people out". The next day I got the letter telling me that I was subversive, and I showed it to Dos. He was infuriated, and determine to do anything he could to clear my name. He said he would write syndicated columns for the best newspapers. There was one other thing that gave me great confidence in friendship.

Hamilton Owens, the Editor of the *Baltimore Sun* and a very wise person, advised me to get the most reactionary people I could find to support me. Owens knew that they would not pay any attention to liberal people. Therefore, he took on the job of recruiting reactionary people, and the most the most important reactionary person found, was a man named Ober, who had introduced a very restrictive bill in the legislature prohibiting anyone who had anything to do with communism from being employed by the state. He persuaded Ober to defend me. Ober managed to it very cleverly. We made up a list of 20 people, some very conservative like William Chamberlain, who would write letters for me substantiating the fact that I had never been interested in communism.

Bill who loved to joke, said, "I was one of the people there wrote a letter for you. Don't you remember?" Dr. Gantt smiled but did not say anything.

Bill: Facetiously said, I was a representative for the anti-conservative group. Gantt ignored this comment.

Gantt: After that happened to me, they found out that Hiss, a person that was respected in Baltimore, was really playing in to the Communists. I thought to myself, "How do these people know, how can they be assured that I am not doing something with the Communists?" The fact, that people, just for pure friendship, were willing to support me, risking their own welfare, really heartened me, almost more than anything else that ever happened in my life. There was one person from the whole list of people that knew me well, who refused to write a letter, and I was very disappointed by his refusal. That really gave me a firm feeling of how your real friends will stick by you in times of need - people like Arnold Rich at Hopkins and Hamilton Owens, and those other people who wrote letters for me substantiating the fact that they had never known me to be subversive.

Pete: Did they accuse you of having bought a teapot in some little communist shop?

Gantt: They said, "You bought things in Maryland Free-state Book Shop." I looked up some literature I had gotten from the Maryland Free-State Book Shop, which might have been run by communists, and I said, "Yes, I did". I remember buying a teapot there."

Ross: So at that time it was communistic to buy a teapot in a liberal bookstore?

Gantt: I remember what Dos Passos said about friendship. He said, "I do not t see why political opinions or any opinions or differences about things should interfere with friendship. I made a list of qualities that I consider the base of friendship. One is tolerance of another person's point of view and opinions. A friend is usually a person you enjoy being with, and a friend is a person who really does not count the cost of standing up for you when you need it. I think friends and friendship are what has meant more to me in my life than almost any other thing."

Gantt: Let me say just one more thing about this: At the same time I was accused of being subversive by the McCarthy group in this country, they published a little pamphlet on me in Russia, which was called "Experimental Neuroses in the USA." They said that although I claimed to be a leader of the Pavlovian group in the US, I was actually very anti-Pavlovian. They said my research work was really designed to support the capitalistic system.

Ross: Because it had a genetic overtone to it, or just a departure from Pavlovian thinking.

Gantt: It was because they wanted to accuse me of anything that they could, in America, of being anti-Pavlovian. It was falling in with the party line to accuse everything outside of Russia was evil. However, I must say that I have had staunch friends in Russia like Bykov. Although I do not go along with all of his scientific work, Bykov never faltered in his friendship toward me. He invited me soon after her was over here for the International Physiological Congress to come and lecture in Russia. The friends I have had have not been confined to one country.

Ross: Was Bykov a member of the Russian parliament?

Gantt: No, well, they do not have any parliament. He was a member of several highly rated scientific committees. He was well thought of by powers in the government of Russia, and he led what was popular in Russia at that time. While we were doing the McCarthy accusations over here, Bykov was also accusing people in Russia of not following Pavlov. Bykov was playing into the government, because Stalin wanted to show that everything that was Russian was better than anything that was not Russian. So the idea was to show that anybody who was Russian was right in their opinion, and that people living in Russia should not quote or say anything nor pay any attention to people who were outside of Russia. That is why they accused me of being anti-Pavlovian. It was just playing into Stalin's political ideas. At the same time, it was interesting that simultaneously while they were accusing me here of being pro-Russian and subversive, they were accusing me in Russia of being anti-Pavlovian, and linked to the capitalists in this country.

Charles Scott Sherrington (1857-1955)

Ross: Who were some of the other people in Europe that you considered friends?

Gantt: I met a number of scientists in Europe such as Sherrington, but I did not know them very well.

Ross: What was Sherrington's reaction to Pavlov's conditioning?

Gantt: He looked on it rather askant and thought Pavlov was wasting his time. He wrote Pavlov that. A Russian sent me a book I found last spring. It had been on my desk for some time, but I hadn't opened it. It was some letters of Pavlov and there was a letter from Sherrington in 1916. Sherrington at that time was in

Liverpool, Professor of Physiology, and he hadn't yet received the Nobel Prize. He wrote to Pavlov asking Pavlov to give him a letter of recommendation for the post of Oxford. Granit, who wrote a biography of Sherrington, was over here last winter. I told him about this letter that Sherrington wrote to Pavlov. He didn't believe it, but I gave him a photostated copy of the letter from the book. So they were friends, but Sherrington kind of took conditional reflex with a grain of salt. I don't think Sherrington understood behavior work. He worked with spinal reflexes.

Bernard Shaw (1856-1950)

Ross: What about Bernard Shaw?

Gantt: I met Bernard Shaw. I would not say that I knew him. I do not know why Shaw was anti-Pavlovian, but he has written a book excoriating Pavlov. Shaw was against the many things. I met him at Lady' Astor is when she tried to get us together. Finally, his t kind of exploded and said, "Well I haven't heard of Pavlov's school, anybody can tell you about a dog secreting saliva".

Ross: Were you able to change his opinion?

Gantt: I do not think I straighten him out, but. He had a sense of humor.

Pete: Did he listen to you?

Gantt: Yes, he would listen. He was a good listener.

Ross: He had a kind of bearlike Pavlov.

Gantt: I said, "Well Mr. Shaw you and Pavlov are very much alike" he kind of chuckled and said,' yes I've heard so." My wife was sitting in between Lord Lothian and Bernard Shaw, and she thought the easier the two to talk to was Lothian, who was an ambassador to this country. Lothian seem to be a little irritated with Gantt's wife and replied saying "Little girl your job is to entertain Mr. Shaw".

Ross: He must have been difficult to entertain.

B. F. Skinner (1904-1990)

Pete: You must have known Skinner pretty well.

Gantt: I had met him at Pavlovian meetings, corresponded with him, and visited him several times in Boston.

Pete: Do you feel like he has made much of a contribution to American psychology?

Gantt: I respect Skinner's honesty. I do not think he has great insight or great intuition. I think Skinner emphasized the external environment, and I do not see that he has added anything to what John B. Watson said.

Ross: Would you say that he was a great operator?

Gantt: I do not think that Skinner conscientiously deceives people, but he had a tremendous facility with words, and he is a very attractive person.

Ross: And he believes what he says?

Gantt: Yes, and people naturally flock to that, and I think Skinner reacts to it. I think Skinner enjoys that kind of adulation and he plays into it.

Ross: This was a facetious play on words in view of Skinner's operant conditioning.

Ross: Do you really think that there is a difference between Pavlovian conditioning and operant conditioning?

Gantt: No, not essentially.

Ross: How do you look at this issue?

Gantt: Well I discussed Pavlovian research with Skinner, including the operant element. For example, I would have the dog open the lid of food can to get the food. I did not do this from the operant viewpoint, because I was only interested in the movements of the dog.

Skinner's operant conditioning was diminished somewhat as a separate entity from other forms of conditioning when two people who had worked with him at Harvard came to Arkansas and started a very successful animal training center of their own (Keller & Marian Breland, 1961). Operant people at that time were inclined to believe that almost anything good could be taught with their methods, including the learning of speech in babies, denying any heredi-tary input. Chomsky's linguistic theory (1964) postulates that the structure of language is biologically determined, in opposition to Skinner's theory of behaviorism. The Breland paper clearly showed what should be taken into account in any type of conditioning. To put it bluntly, a duck cannot run like a rabbit, and a rabbit cannot swim or quack like a duck. So for success in conditioning, it is nec-essary to take into account inborn reflexes of the animal you have chosen for your research, including age, sex, health, and other char-acteristics. Lorenz (1950) and Tinbergen (1951) argued that when you plan research on any animal, you should first study its instinctive behaviors. In his early publications, Pavlov (1922, 1923) argued that instincts could be better understood as reflexes, and there is no need for the term instinct. Pavlov said, "whatever they are called, they are responses of the organism to internal and external stimuli (pp. 9-11 in the Anrep translation)."

Ogden Nash (1902-1971)

Pete: What was your relation with Ogden Nash?

Gantt: Yes, I knew Ogden Nash fairly well. He visited my house especially during the last two years of his life. He wrote in a book, "Inscribed for Horsley, politely not coarsely. I am tired of bores..." Then, I for-gotten the last time I asked him how he decided to go into poetry, so I asked him again. He said, "Well I had been interested in writ-ing poetry when I was a youth and since I couldn't be a great poet, I would rather be a good bad poet than a bad good poet."

Henry Louis Mencken "H. L. Mencken" (1880-1956)

Ross: I remember you telling me that you knew Mencken. What was he like?

Gantt: I have met people over here such as Mencken, known for their literacy. Mencken lived in Baltimore. I knew Fitzgerald pretty well and met other people such as Sinclair Lewis. A good friend of mine, Maurice Hindus, wrote a good deal about Russia. I saw a good deal of Mencken when he was in Baltimore. We were both members of the Hamilton Street Men's Club. He was rather shy and he did not like crowds. He liked that small intimate group.

Ross: What was his behavior in groups?

Gantt: He was rather cynical and satirical. He usually enjoyed making fun of things. During the Depression some religious radical liberal group at leftist college in Oklahoma, wrote to Mencken for a contribution. Mencken wrote them back, and said he was sorry he could not give them money, but he would pray for them.

Ross: When I was working with you, we frequently discussed different types of conditioning. Hilgard made a distinction between classical conditioning, which was Pavlovian conditioning, and instrumental conditioning, which was more in the tradition of Bechterev and Thorndike. I remember you thinking that this was a rather inappropriate term. That is, Pavlov studied both kinds of conditioning and it was wrong to assume that Pavlov did just one kind of conditioning.

Gantt: Yes, Pavlov in having the dog break the current when he lifted his leg did what they considered operant conditioning. Pavlov used that method.

Ross: Do you think classical conditioning is a good term?

Gantt: Well I never used it, but I sometimes use it now. I really do not see the justification for making rigid categories. I think you should describe the method you are using, but whether to consider one extremely different from another on that basis is another thing. Some of the Russians do not think there is a difference (Asratyan (1972), Kupaalov (1949) & Rabinovich, (1955). The last author and others have done experiments, in which the electrical activity (EEG) of the brain, was used as reinforced signals.

Ross: I would like to turn now to your research and to the people that have at worked with you.

Gant: Well you are qualified to talk about this since you are one of my chief research collaborators beginning in 1950.

Ross: I did my most significant research work when I was working with you, and it influenced everything I did after I left Hopkins.

Gantt: Perhaps one of the most important projects to come out of the laboratory was your study showing that the heart rate and blood pressure conditional responses were proportional to the unconditional stimulus intensity. The blood pressure work was particularly important. It was the first to show the effect of both excitatory and inhibitory conditional stimuli. Another important point that came out of your research was the retention of the heart rate and blood pressure conditional responses over 13 month period with no further reinforcement.

Ross: Yes, was interesting that the differentiated CR in four dogs was larger than it was when the experiment was temporarily halted. In talking with medical students and other people, I was always impressed with their reluctance to accept Pavlov's research as important.

Gantt: Apparently, physiologists recognized mainly his work on digestion. However, that was a long time ago, and it is almost forgotten. For his work on digestion in 1903, he received the first Nobel Prize in physiology in 1904. Since then, Pavlov was then known chiefly for his work on conditional reflexes. However, in many physiological textbooks, there may be a section on conditional reflexes, but no referenced Pavlov.

Ross: What do you think of this?

Gantt: It probably results from a very strong school of behavioral psychology in America. They have gone back to their own roots, which came down through Thorndike, Watson, and Skinner. This was looked on by the American behaviors as a different branch of the conditioning tree. It had taken a different turn, they either do not want or did not see the connection with the early basic Pavlovian research. I think many of the psychologists, certainly Skinner, recognizes the importance of Pavlov. However, many of them, who are less historically minded just consider, these Americans thought that Pavlov did this work many years ago, and that's all past history, and now we're going to do something new and different. You are closer to psychology. What do you think of this opinion?

Ross: I do not know. I have tried to think about the difference between the two approaches, the Pavlovian approach and the traditional American psychological approach. One seems to emphasize that whatever is reinforced will be learned, and that is an excellent way of shaping behavior. The other, the Pavlovian empathizes pairing: things that get together stay together (recent research on pairing shows that it is extremely important). Whenever Pavlovian researchers use the term reinforcement, it is generally just a synonym for pairing.

Gantt: Pavlov in 1922 acknowledged Thorndike as the creator of the conditional reflex construct in his work on animal intelligence in 1898. Pavlov also spoke about Watson, saying there was a very different approach to the subject of conditioning between the Americans and him. He said the Americans were always looking for the practical applications of conditioning. Pavlov was more interested in physiology. I think that still characterizes the two schools. Americans want something that will quickly get results. Skinner obtains his results in many ways. It is a quickly applicable method, I think. Recently, some Americans are trying to use the Pavlovian method. What do they want? They want a method that will quickly cure heart disease, and that will modify all of the viscera. They have neglected do what Pavlov did, to first study the laws of visceral functions. They rush out and say how they modify heart rate and blood pressure. The same difference exists now as Pavlov pointed out in his 1922 book. People like Neal Miller and his school very much want to modify renal function, cardiac function, and of course they're looking for the Messiah – and they can't wait for a careful study of the basic laws.

Ross: When you explain in detail to medical students the salivary research of Pavlov, they say, "So what." They overlook the fact that the salivary conditional response is a very complex autonomic response, and can be altered by any stimulus such as the site of a stranger. After a bit of talking, some of them see its importance as illustrating some of the basic principles of neurophysiology including the excitatory and inhibitory effects of neurotransmitters. I think it's important to remember that all of Pavlov's fundamental concepts were based on the actions of neurons of wires that connect the different parts of the brain with each other.

Gantt: The neurotransmitter research came very much later, long after Pavlov died. Otto Loewi, a German born pharmacologist won the Nobel Prize in Physiology of Medicine in 1936, which he shared with a friend Sir Henry Dale. He is been thought of as the Father of Neuroscience. Pavlov died in 1936 so he knew nothing about chemical transmission at synapses, which gives his series of excitation and inhibition a more solid ground. Acetylcholine was a neurotransmitter that Loewi discovered. When this substance is secreted by the Vegas nerve, heart rate is slowed very quickly, Dykman in Gantt 1959) investigated the action of the Vegas nerve on heart rate CRs. Dogs were given large doses of atropine, known to completely block vagal action (Salman, 1948). Digitized heart rate has two components in dogs, an initial component of deceleration and a subsequent component of acceleration. The slowdown component is mediated by the vague and the acceleration component by adrenalin secreted by the kidneys stimulating the sympathetic nervous system. Atropine removed the very quick slow down reflex part of the conditioned wave, leaving the later sympathetic reflex intact. Removal of the vagal input (the brake on the heart), rapidly increases heart rate acceleration.

Pavlov considered salivation simply a method of quantitative measurement. It was simply a kind of yardstick, and it was not just salivation to the signal for food. Pavlov was interested in what you could do with this method in discovering the basis of cerebral action.

Ross: It is important to recognize that the salivary research of Pavlov was the earliest study of autonomic conditioning. It is just as important to look at salvation as it is heart rate in discovering new laws.

Gantt: It has been 72 years since Pavlov described the conditional reflex. At that time he was 36 years old. He died 36 years later in 1936. Much of the work that has come after him simply asked the same question that Pavlov asked in the beginning of his research. "What question you asked of nature is very important in science." That at is what opens up a new field. Pavlov asked the fundamental question: "How can an autonomic function be modified by the external environment, and how can it be measured." Now that is an important question. Pavlov began with certain ideas which were largely from the current neurophysiology, but he modified his ideas considerably on the basis of the observations he made. If you analyze what has been done since Pavlov's death you'll find in many other people, even though studying autonomic function, are still asking the same question that Pavlov asked: "Can the autonomic function be modified by the external environment"? They are not asking a new question. What they are doing is giving various elaborations of that same question that Pavlov put to nature. They may be defining the question in a more detailed way, and this might be important. They are, however, stereotyped in that they are not asking any new question. They're not pioneers in the sense that Pavlov was.

Ross: Let us talk for a few minutes about your early work when you first came to this country, and started the Pavlovian laboratory. What were the things you concentrated on the immediately?

Gantt: I too began with the study of two drugs, Amytal and caffeine.

Ross: Did this sort of open the field psychopharmacology?

Gantt: I don't know that it open it up. I worked on drugs off and on throughout. I came to Hopkins in 1929, that's roughly 43 years ago. I was very much interested in some of the quantitative relationships between the conditional reflex and the unconditional stimulus, and I did what Pavlov had not done: I measured the amount of salivary secretion to the amount of food that was given, and obtain curves for both the conditional reflex and the unconditional reflex. It's amazing how even some very important things remain untouched, not worked on by Pavlov, who focused on the relationship of the conditional reflex to the unconditional stimulus, which is a linear relationship discovered by Gantt.

Ross: As I understand it from reading one of your later books, Experimental Basis for Neurotic Behavior, Gantt (1944), you studied two different mathematical relations: first the intensity of the conditional stimulus on the CR which is exponential in form; and second the intensity of the unconditional stimulus or the CR which is linear.

Gantt: The exponential function that Gantt discovered imply that the intensity of the CS may be more important in determining the magnitude of the CR than the UCS. (My interpretation now. I did not discuss with Dr. Gantt). Also, as I mentioned above, it is possible to turn a UCS into a CS. When dogs fight or food, they frequently suffer injuries, which is a relatively strong UCS, but not strong enough to extinguish the food reflex. In this case, the defensive reflex becomes a CS, which when paired with the UCS food produces the CR.

Ross: What were your first studies on heart rate?

Gantt: In the 1930's I became interested in heart rate. I was interested in how heart rate changes with the intensity of the conditional stimulus. Although cardiac changes were not in the sense an issue; they were worked on at the time I published the first paper in 1940 with Hoffman, a very good physiologists who came to work with me from Norway. He said when he first arrived in 1939 that he did not want to work on this problem, because he did not believe there would be any changes, but I persuaded him to work on this, and we found very definite respiratory and cardiac changes. The other problem I desired to solve was that of identifying the parts of a reflex arc that are involved in the formation of the conditional reflex.

Ross: Actually, that work began before the cardiac work, didn't it?

Gantt: Yes, it began in 1932.

Ross: You got into four fields: one was the laws of conditioning having to do with the intensity of the conditional stimulus and the unconditional stimulus; the second the psychopharmacological research, the third the neurophysiological work attempting to find out the role that the brain plays in conditioning; and the fourth heart rate conditioning. Let's go back to the central parts of the reflex are. What were the main findings of that research?

Gantt: There is one more field I should mention because it began early and went on for 15 to 20 years, and is still going on many places. During 1930 to 1942, Loucks & I were studying conditioning and differentiation. An important discovery was made that didn't have anything to do with the research. We found that one of the three dogs (Nick) developed an experimental neurosis. He eventually became better known in many countries than I. Over a period of many years, he developed many new neurotic behaviors, not present at first. These new behaviors spontaneously emerged throughout his life, so I got into experimental neurosis in the '30s' through the side door.

Ross: And you actually studied heart rate changes at that time?

Gantt: Yes. I studied heart rate changes as part of the experimental neurosis, and although I studied many neurotic dogs, I've never intentionally produced a neurotic state in a dog. Always, the neurotic right state occurred in one "nervous or excitable dog" and not others.

Ross: The conclusion appears to be that dogs become neurotic, if and only if, they are predisposed to become neurotic. Is that what you're saying?

Gantt: It is probably a genetic factor. The development of a neurosis depends upon the type of dog more than the events they experience.

Ross: Do not think that the experiences that dogs have in painful conditioning procedures or dogfights or any other type of abuse they accidentally receive can produce an experimental neurosis?

Gantt: Not unless you have that type of excitable dog that is predisposed to react negatively to stress. Pavlov thought you could produce an experimental neurosis by difficult discrimination between excitatory and inhibitory stimuli. I show that this is more a matter of the type of dog than a conflict between excitation and inhibition.

Ross: Did Pavlov recognize that the type of dog was very important?

Gantt: Yes after the flood in Leningrad in 1924, he said that type is important, but he still thought that the most important thing was a conflict between excitation and inhibition. He did not appreciate the importance of the exponential relationship between the CS and the UCS.

DYKMAN & GANTT, (1960) wrote a paper describing an experimental neurosis in an excitable male dog (Schnapps) that was produced accidentally by a high voltage shock (120 volts, 60 Hz, AC). The actual accident occurred in 1950, and at that time I was only interested in saving the dog (Schnapps) for the research I was doing on cardiac conditioning and differentiation (Dykman, Gantt, & Whitehorn, 1956). The published papers were based on research completed in 1951. For details of the experiment the reader should consult the original 1960 paper.

The conditional stimuli that used in most conditioning experiments elicit the OR, and are generally desirable to extinguish the OR before initiating the reinforcement procedure. In the OR phase in the autonomic study mentioned above, dogs were given 5 to 15 repetitions of each of the three non-reinforcement tones/day. Each of four dogs had been habituated to the conditioning stand, and had received over 250 repetitions of tones as ORs with no electrical stimulation. Hence, the OR was partially extinguished before they received any electrical stimulation. Pavlov gradually came to view the OR as an important response and in 1916, discussed inquisitiveness as an elaboration of the OR.

I had purchased a Variac to regulate voltage. Unfortunately, I found out in working with Schnapps, the first animal to be electrically stimulated after the OR was partially extinguished, that the electrical cord connecting the Variac could be plugged into the wall circuit in two ways, one of which delivered a high-voltage shock. I solved this problem in a few days by inserting a step down and step up transformer into the circuit that powered the Variac. At that time, few buildings had grounded wall plugs. Also, we didn't have enough money to buy an expensive electrical stimulator.

The purpose of this experiment was to compare both the cardiac and motor components of entered the OR. Each dog received only three electrical stimuli that were never paired with the tones that were used to generate the OR, part of the pre-conditioning sensitization test in the original experiment.

Each UCS lasted from 2 to 5 seconds and the interval between was approximately 5 minutes. While the current was applied was applied to the left front leg, it irradiated to the heart rate leads located on the chest. Each of the three electrical stimuli produced an immediate withdrawal reaction. The duration of the struggling increased for about five minutes following the third shock. I entered the conditioning chamber after each electrical stimulus, attempting to determine the source of the difficulty. By the third stimulus the dog was frantic: his heart rate had increased to about 190 bpm. He was struggling in an attempt to get out of the stand, and had moved as far back as possible in an attempt to escape the shock.

He urinated, defecated, and vomited; a sexual erection was noted following the third shock. Also, the dog refused to eat after he was removed from the conditioning stand.

On the day following the orienting resume without electrical stimulation. Schnapps was more restless than usual. The motoric actions of the OR were exaggerated, heart rate was substantially increased, and he refused to eat when he was taken back to the kennels. His behavior was interpreted as a mild upset, and the striking changes that followed were not expected. During the next 24 days, most of the behaviors produced by the electric shocks shops gradually returned. New behaviors also appeared. A muscular tremor developed in the upper muscles of the leg that been shocked on the 12th day. On the 18th day following shock, Schnapps exhibited signs of fear on seeing me and the animal caretaker. He crouched in the corner of the kennel with his tail between his legs. The animal refused to come to the experimental room on the 22nd day by walking with me down the stairs, but showed no hesitation about entering the elevator. Normally, the animals were brought to the experimental room in the basement in the elevator, but when it was busy we used the stairs.

During the 24-day period during which these pathological symptoms appear and intensified, numerous attempts were made to extinguish them extra care walks with the experimenter, special foods and dog treats. Multiple daily sessions were run, and experiments were conducted with the door to the conditioning room open. Schnapps was even moved to another conditioning chamber one day to see if this would help. None of this changed his fearfulness.

I decided one day that I should try desensitization, what Whitehorn had referred to as reassurance of mildness (Whitehorn, 1953). The shock intensity was set at a level that would just produce noticeable muscle twitch. Schnapps received 15 mild shocks the first day of treatment and 20 mild shocks the next day. All of these symptoms gradually disappeared except for his persistence in wanting to go the conditioning room by the way of the elevator rather than the stairs. He struggled violently when I attempted to get him to walk down the stairs with me.

Ross: It seems to me that the term experimental neurosis is it an in-
        valid descriptor. Neuroses occur in certain types of dogs, who
        like many humans, overreact to the everyday stresses of life –
        stresses barely perceptible to stable dogs and humans. It is a le-
        gitimate neurosis, but not an experimental neurosis. The cause
        lies in the genes passed onto individuals from their parents.

Gantt: That is interesting, and it may be a more acceptable way of en-
        couraging people to think about the causes of neurosis.

Dawkins (2009) reports a very interesting experiment by Penny, Foulds, &
Hendy (1982). They constructed a genetic tree from five different proteins
sequences. The five proteins were those for hemoglobin Amend, hemoglobin B (hemoglobin's are important in oxygen uptake in blood cells),
fibrinopeptide A, and fibrinopeptide B (clot blood), and cytochrome C
(important in cellular biochemistry). These five substances can be found
in all species, but they vary in amount in different species. According
to Dawkins, these proteins can be looked at in 34 million different ways
in assessing evolutionary change. Penny et al devised a tree diagram
which showed the interrelations of common domestic animals in the top
branches, and the relations of chimpanzees and monkeys to humans in
the lower branches. The upper diagram indicated that the cow and dog
were closer related in DNA with both of these species related more remotely to the pig. The horse was next entered and was closely related
to the three just named (a total of 4 species at this point). The dog was a
last species enter the top part of the diagram (now 5 distinct evolutionary species). It is interesting that my tiny Chihuahua and his much larger
friend a standard poodle are both descended from wolves, all dogs are
descended from wolves. Humans have created the different breeds by
selecting breeding. The most interesting part of the tree included those
branches demonstrating a close relation between humans and chimpanzees, supposedly sharing some 98% of their DNA. The rhesus monkey
was related to both the human and chimpanzee but more remotely. The
rabbit came next with the kangaroo family having less DNA in common

with humans than any other species in the branches of the lower tree. Penny described 11 different species of animals, and had apparently analyzing a huge number of different combinations of animals to come up with these 11 species. This ingenious research might eventually make it possible to describe the interrelations of DNA in all species – the fish and turtles in the oceans and freshwaters, birds wherever they live. It appears to me that a comparison of shared gene estimates with those of shared DNA in humans or any other species in which these estimates have been made, that DNA is more sensitive metric in assessing species differences than gene count.

Robert W. Doty (1920-2011)

Doty introduces his chapter, saying,

> "Above all, Horsley Gant was a disciple of Ivan Petrovich Pavlov. One deliberately uses the word 'disciple', for such was a remarkable force of Pavlov's personality and ideas, that essentially all of the students who attained distinction did so by following with faithfulness uncommon in science, the methodology and precepts of the master.
>
> Gantt's beginnings with Pavlov follow the same procedure as Babkin (1949) for the era some 20 or more years earlier. First, the initiate was given a minor problem, the results of which would be largely confirmatory of work previously done in the laboratory. In Gantt's case, this was establishing the fact that a dog stomach produces 2=3 times as much secretion when black bread is introduced into the fistula, as one white bread is used (Gant, 1924). Next was a study with Kupalov comparing external pancreatic secretion induced by cut versus chopped meat (Gantt and Kupalov, 1927). Both of these studies appeared in German.

However, these early studies also already testified to one of Gantt's major scientific endeavors, to bring the fruits of knowledge gained in the laboratory to bear upon the problems of the clinic. Witness as he was to the appalling deprivation wrought throughout Russia by war and two revolutions, where up to 11 million people were at one time served by relief agencies of Great Britain and the United States. Even as his armies invaded the country, epidemics were rife, 50% of the people were illiterate (Gantt, 1924 1936). Gantt was ever after empathetic to the potential misery of human beings in his frequent source of ignorance. Much of Gantt's thought and work was as directed toward applying science to practical medical ends, but I leave the development of this theme to other contributions of this volume."

Of particular significant to Gantt's major career was a publication of the paper in Brain, as it marked the beginning of his dedication to making the work of the Pavlovian school accessible to the English-speaking world. This was the result in the publication of several reviews (Gantt. 1927, 1932, &1970), the translation of major tracks by Pavlov (1928 &194), and (Gantt, Pickenhain, & Zwingmann, 1970).

Completes work, were in justified, in the era 1903 – 1920, and while the work with Pavlov was doing seemed interesting, those lacking access to the Russian literature did not know quite what it was. Lasley noted in 1913 – 1914 the accumulated of a list of 300 papers on conditional reflexes, only seven of which can be found in major American libraries (Babkin, 1940 & Orbach (ed.) Neurophysiology after Lasley, pp.1 – 20, 1982. Pavlov, himself, was distinctly not helpful. Between 1903 in 1920, essentially only four accounts were published by Pavlov in Western Europe concerning his work on conditional reflexes… Beritashvili in Brain finally provided a thorough, critical review of much of the Pavlovian work, complete with methodology, new data, and any references *available to world literature. This placed this line of research fully in the current framework of neurophysiological investigation."* *(McGuigan/Ban, 1955).*

It was obvious in reading this chapter that Doty was far more impressed with Gantt than he was with Pavlov. Gantt took on a different track than Pavlov did when establishing his own laboratory at John Hopkins. Pavlov won a Nobel Prize, and Gantt was nominated for it. Gantt remained loyal to the founder, Pavlov. Doty admits in writing this chapter about Gantt that he had been following Gantt's career very closely in his early studies. He wrote a very good summary of the work of one of Gantt's students, Roger Brown Loucks. Doty refers to Loucks as an extremely capable electrical engineer, who while working in Gantt's laboratory in 1933, wrote the criticism of Pavlov's theory of irradiation. After Pavlov discovered inhibition and excitation, he postulated that these effects could spread to other parts of the brain. The easiest situation for demonstrating innovation excitation, as I said above is to present two conditional stimuli, one which is reinforced on every trial and the other which is not reinforced on any trial. In the case of the motor response (flexion), differentiation occurs rapidly when the unconditional stimulus is an electrical stimulation of one of the legs. In the case of heart rate conditioning, and undifferentiated response appears sometimes after only one trial in which the conditional stimulus is paired with the unconditional electrical stimulus, but differentiation develops more slowly than it does where the motor response. In fact, I have never seen a complete extinction of the heart rate response to the negative conditional stimulus, the one not reinforced. But there is a huge difference between the one that is reinforced and the one that is not reinforced in terms of the differential effects on heart rate. Pavlov's concept of a radiation simply assumes that either the innovation process or the excitation process spreads to different areas of the cortex.

Loucks (1933) said that the data to support irradiation concept were insufficient, and in fact, contradictory to what Pavlov claimed. Doty says,

> "One does not know Gantt's role or reaction in this, we're just the previous year, he written of five – page summary (Gantt, 1932) in which the fanciful inferences on cortical activity were included without reservation, and even as late in as 1948 in his article for the 'Annual Review of Physiology' he avoided any mention of this debate. I knew from working with him, that he was very skeptical of anything that could not be verified repeatedly. Doty wrote his chapter in 1955, and the major work on neurotransmitters began in the 1980's, and is still going on. These neurotransmitters do spread to different cortical areas. The two that were most important in widespread transmission are classified as ionotropic receptors (Scabo, Gould, & Manji, 2000). Most relevant to the present discussion is the following quote on p.5), which suggests that Pavlov's concept of irradiation is now backed up by neural transmitter research."

Often, the ionotropic receptors can be composed of different compositions of the different subunits, thereby providing the system with considerable flexibility. For example, there is extensive research into the potential development of an anxiolytic that is devoid of sedative effects by targeting $GABA_A$ receptor subunits present in selected brain regions. In general, neurotransmission that is mediated by ionotropic receptors is very fast, with ion channels opening and closing within milliseconds, and these regulates much of the tonic excitatory (i.e., glutamate – mediated) and inhibitory (i.e., GABA – mediated) activity in the CNS: we discuss below many of the classical neurotransmitters (e.g., momoamines) exert their effects on a short timescale, and are therefore often considered to be modulatory in their effects.

John Lacey (1915-2004)

Lacey (1956) wrote a paper for the Annals of New York Academy of Sciences entitled *The Evaluation of Autonomic Responses –Toward a General Solution.* He provides a thorough review of the scientific literature on autonomic conditioning without going into details for much of the quoted work. For example, in discussing Haggard (1949) he did not quote what Haggard said. Haggard studied 50 boys and 50 girls, 17 years of age. Each participant responded ton a2500 words, assessed by four GSR measures. These included SR changes, conductance changes, log resistance changes and log conductance changes. Log conductance changes best satisfied the criteria of additivity, homogeneity of variance, independence of means and variances, randomness, and maximal precision. He was apparently unaware that Wilder (1950, 1957) found autonomic responses (not just skin resistance or skin conductance) inversely related to the magnitude of prestimulus levels of functioning. Lacey claims that the numerous transformations made on autonomic responses ignore physiological processes, namely the law of initial values (Wilder), and basic physiology homeostatic processes. It is difficult for me to see why the analysis of Haggard necessarily ignores physiological mechanisms. It has all desirable features one would like to find in any statistical analysis of data of skin conductance data, the only autonomic response he observed. From what Haggard said, I assume that had he been analyzing heart rate and skin conductance at the same time, he would have analyzed them separately.

Autonomic functioning at resting levels is nearly always very high for SR in normally healthy adults and children but just a few beats up or down for HR, with small changes upward in both diastolic and systolic blood pressure (BP). We followed Lacey in the beginning of our statistical analyses, first removing the regression of stimulus levels on prestimulus levels, and then computing T-scores with a mean of 50 and a standard error (SE) of 10. T-scores were the normalized using methods described by Crocker & Algina (2006). It turns out that there is an easy way to do this that is not used by psycho-physiologists in constructing moving averages. Tamhane & Dunlap (2000) describe a technique that can be used to summarize time series data (data that arise in the series presentation of stimuli). Two types of sequences or averages can be computed: moving averages and exponentially weighted moving averages. Stationary trends can be modeled using regression techniques (linear trend fitted by a straight-line). The model maps dependence between successive observations. More advanced techniques are proposed by Box and Jenkins 1976. But in working with correlations, it is easy to make directional changes in two different autonomic systems the same without altering the magnitude of the correlations or size of responses. It is true that the magnitude of changes in each autonomic system is related to the prestimulus level (p. 126 in the Lacey paper). This is not a problem when one variable can be correctly labeled as dependent upon another.

Lacey suggests that investigators of autonomic function have used a large number of transformations that are not rooted in physiological factor theory. This certainly does not apply to Haggard who focused exclusively on one autonomic measure (log of skin conductance). Lacey states that he is seeking a theory that applies to all autonomic measures, but he does not consider responses of internal organs such as the kidney, sweat glands, salivary glands, Anrep on Pavlov (1927), Darrow (1934, & 1937), Stevens (1951), Stevens & Galanter (1957), and Gantt (1944).

Lacey backs up his theory by an intensive review of the physiological research most of which appeared in physiological textbooks written in 1940, and in specific papers that he lists. He begins his discussion in a paragraph (p. 127) labeled *Homeostatic restraints of response.* He writes as follows:

"A large number of experimental observations suggest that any induced excitation or inhibition of an autonomically innervated structure instantly initiates a series of changes that serve to mollify the disturbance... The corollary is this, the record of autonomic response is a function of both the induced magnitude of

autonomic activation (as would be seen in the absence of contrary changes) and of the promptness and vigor of secondarily induced autonomic changes that serve to restrain and limit the effects of the initial disturbance."

The last sentence in the quote is crucial in that the changes that serve to restrain the effects of the initial disturbance are far more restrictive in some autonomic functions than in others. I have already alluded to this in discussing HR and SR. Lacey states that all autonomic responses are controlled by homeostatic mechanisms. While this is true, it is only a part of the story. Gantt (1944) demonstrated in many experiments that homeostatic mechanisms can be completely submerged by conditions which lead to the production unexpected responses, and this happens often. The analysis that Lacey did gave him no chance to see that homeostasis is insufficient to account for the discrepancies in system differences that occur in autonomic functioning. Gantt added the principle of schizokinesis to account for the fact that while each organ normally does its own thing in the domain of homeostatic processes, it fails for example, to account for the fact that the urine flow of the kidney is greatly inhibited by previous experiences of stress, while heart rate is increased by stress. The kidney response was an unexpected response; the expected normal homeostatic response occurred back in the kennels. The dogs in the Dykman et al. study described above produced zero urine flow for over an hour when placed in a room in which they had previously received electrical stimulation, but emptied their bladders immediately upon being returned to their home cages. As said above, we had filled their stomachs with water using a stomach tube prior to bringing them to the conditioning room. The retention of urine in the conditioning room was not expected. Why should the kidneys shut down and not continue to secrete urine? This was not just a simple matter of retention of urine in the bladder, since the urine created by the kidneys could not reach the bladder. The tubes that normally connect to the bladder had previously been surgically disconnected from the bladder, and moved to an exterior body surface. Thus, we could immediately detect any secretion produced by the kidneys. This is a nice example of Gantt's principle of schizokinesis, in which a normal homeostatic reaction is overridden by a previously established conditional emotional response.

Autokinesis, described above, is related in which new unexpected normal or pathological behaviors develop over time following a trauma or more simply the inability to adapt to the everyday experiences of life. This occurs in dogs that have a nervous temperament. The dog, and I suppose humans, suddenly decide that they want to do something different, after doing the same thing for months. No experimental condition is changed – yet some new behavior not expected emerges. One of our dogs (Schnaps as described above), after experiencing just one intense electrical stimulus (by accident), which we treated successfully by giving him a series of barely perceptible electrical stimuli to desensitize his fears, would no longer walk down the stairs to the conditioning room. He persisted in dragging the animal caretaker or me to the elevator, which we occasionally used prior to his unfortunate experience. Most often, the dog ran 'happily with us' down six flights of stairs to the conditioning room. Gantt cites many evidences of this in following the spontaneous development of pathological changes in the behavior of Nick, a dog that he observed for several years (see Gantt, 1944). Nick had developed an experimental neurosis spontaneously without ever exposed to any painful stimulus. Again, one of those dogs could not tolerate stresses and strains of these everyday experiences.

When you analyze skin resistance and compare with heart rate, you see huge system differences. As Singer & Willett (2003) said. "When researchers get caught up in the novel and complex analysis, they often need to be reminded just what is this is to a statistical model is and what it is not." Now, SR or the older term GSR is an entirely different kind of response from HR and systolic and diastolic blood pressure. Both are important to survival but in entirely different ways. I was taught in an undergraduate physiology course that sweating is controlled by a parasympathetic output from the sympathetic nervous system. It seemed strange to that the sympathetic nervous system (so-called, flight and fight system) system contained parasympathetic output (cholinergic nerve tracts). Shibasaki & Crandall (2011) review the scientific studies of sweating in humans. The paper reviews the important research of Nadal and colleagues. Nadal et al write as follows:

"With the understanding that internal and mean skin temperatures both have the capability to control sweating, researchers began to assess the relationship between contributions of skin do internal temperature in the modulation of sweat rate. Early in the 1970's, 'Nadal et al.' Performed seminal work in this area during 'dynamic' increases in internal temperature in humans. The question of the influence of internal and skin temperatures governing sweating was further addressed in non-human primates in which direct measures of brain temperature were obtained. These studies concluded that sweating is primarily controlled by brain temperature, and secondarily modulated by mean skin temperature, which is generally the current consensus of the scientific community.

The primary thermal regulatory center, first reported in the late 1800's, is located within the pre-optic hypothalamic regions of the brain. Because of the difficulty of precisely defining neural pathways responsibility for sweating, in humans, these pathways are not entirely understood. Based upon evidence from animal studies and human anatomical data, the neural pathways from the brain to sweat glands is thought to be as follows: different signals from the pre-optic hypothalamus travel via the tegmentum of pons in the medullary raphe regions to the interinomediolateral column of the spinal cord. Neurons emerge from the ventral horn, passed through the white ramus communicans, combined with peripheral nerves and traveled the sweat glands, with these nerve fibers 'entwined round' the paragrandular tissue of the ecrine sweat glands."

The sympathetic nerve distributed to sweat glands consists of large number cholinergic terminals and a few adrenergic terminals. The effect of the adrenergic terminals causing sweating is minimal given that exogenous administration of adrenergic agents will cause only minimal sweating relative to acetylcholine administration, the latter. The latter the primary neurotransmitter of sweating administration of atropine (a muscarinic receptor antagonist) greatly attenuates or abolishes sweating during a verbal challenge for doing exogenous administration of acetylcholine or its analogs, further confirming that dominance of the cholinergic system and muscarinic receptors in human sweating. Those interested in the physiology of sweat, and its physical and central connections should read this article. Here, I have only summarized some of its important sections, those of most interest to myself and collaborators because of the work we did on the sweat glands and the GSR (Juniper *et al.*). It is obvious, when you look at the literature on sweating and the activation of sweat glands that the GSR response including sweat gland activation is different from that for cardiovascular responses. The serial effects of stimuli dominate GSR, exhausting it in successive repetitions of stimuli within sessions and over days. All that seems to matter is whatever occurs first, whether emotional stimuli or just simple tones. Tones can override powerful emotionally stimuli if they occur first in time. Cardiovascular responses are protected from overreacting by hypothalamic nuclei. These circuits ensure that cardiovascular functions will always room to respond to some new emergency. Given this, one wonders whether one should even attempt to scale GSR's and cardiovascular reactions on the same scale. Darrow (1927) emphasized the independence of skin conductance cardiovascular activity. We have come to the conclusion that he was correct. Of course, Lacey and we have analyzed these functions separately. Once the stimulus and prestimulus levels are separately linearized, you can theoretically compare them with each other -by transforming the results to T-scores. These are generally horribly skewed, but this can be corrected to some extent by various normalization procedures. But is it right to take two systems with vastly different physiological properties and assume that you have accurate measures of both? I say no! I suggest that the very large differences between the GSR and cardiovascular functions should be attributed to schizogenesis and not to manipulations of T or Z scores. GSRs are a more sensitive measure then heart rate or blood pressure in revealing differences in autonomic functioning in humans or dogs, and likely in all warm-blooded species. Heart rate and blood pressure (especially systolic are vastly different kinds of measures than skin conductance, as we pointed out above, serving critical physiological processes related to survival. SR generally drops 50,000 of ohms or more with any novel stimulus; the largest response is to the stimulus that occurs first in time, whether emotional or non-emotional. While heart rate and blood pressure move up or down with noel stimuli as was discussed above; (e.g. up with mental arithmetic and down with novel tones. It is my opinion, that it it is wrong to use standardized regression scores, as Lacey and Lacey did in (1958) to devise a method inn which all autonomic functions can be reliably compared with each other Each physiological function should be s analyzed separately when it is obvious that they are different from each other. The arithmetic should coincide with the physiology and not in any other way.

References

Adams, T. (1966). Characteristics of eccrine sweat gland activity in the footpad of the cat. *Journal of Applied Physiology, 21, 1004-1012.*

Adams, T., & Vaughn, J. A. (1965). Human eccrine sweat gland activity and palmar electrical resistance. *Journal of Applied Physiology, 20,980-983.*

Andreason, N. C. (2014, July). Secrets of the creative brain. *Atlantic Monthly, 313(6), 62.*

Anrep, G. V., & Pavlov, I. P. (1960). *Conditioned reflexes: An investigation of the physiological activity of the cerebral cortex.* New York: Dover Publications.

Aserinsky, E. (1996). The discovery of REM sleep. *Journal of the History of Neurosciences, 5, 213-227.*

Aserinsky, E., & Kleitman, N. (1953). Regularly occurring periods of eye motility and concomitant phenomena during sleep. *Science Magazine, 118, 273-275.*

Aserinksy, E., & Kleitman, N. (1955). Two types of ocular motility occurring during sleep. *Journal of Applied Physiology, 8, 1-10.*

Asratyan, E. A. (1972). Conditional reflex theory and motivational behavior. *Institute of Higher Nervous Activity and Neurophysiology.* Moscow, USSR.

Benjamin, A. T. (2011). *The Secrets of mental math.* Chantilly, Virginia: The Great Courses.

Bitterman, M. E., & Holtzman, W. H. (1952). A factorial study of adjustment to stress. *The Journal of Abnormal and Social Psychology, 52(2), 179-185.*

Box, G. E. P., & Jenkins, G. M. (1976). *Time Series Analysis: Forecasting and Control.* San Francisco: Holden-Day.

Breland, K., & Breland, M. (1961). The misbehavior of organisms. *American Psychologist, 16,681-684.*

Buettner, K. J. K. (1959). Diffusion of water vapor through small areas of human skin in a normal environment. *Journal of Applied Physiology, 14, 269-275.*

Buettner, K. J. K, & Odland, G. F. (1957). Physical factors of the skin barrier layer and water diffusion into human skin. *Fed. Proc., 16, 18, (abstract).*

Cautela, J. R. (1987). The problem of backward conditioning: revisited. In F. J. McGuigan, & T. A. Ban (Eds.), *Critical issues in psychology, psychiatry, and physiology (pp. 149-164).* New York: Gordon and Breach Science Publishers.

Chomsky, N. (1964). The logical basis of linguistic theory. *Preprints of the ninth International Congress of Linguists.*

Corah, N. L., & Stern, J. A. (1963). Stability and adaptation of some measures of electrodermal activity in children. *Journal of experimental Psychology, 65, 80-85.*

Coles, M.G.H., Jennings, J.R., Stern, J.A. (Eds.). (1984). *Psychophysiological perspectives: Festschrift for Beatrice and John Lacey.* New York: Van Nostrand Reinhold Company Inc.

Connors, CK. (1969). A teacher rating scale for use in drug studies with children. *American Journal of Psychiatry, 126, 884-888.*

Crocker, L. M., & Algina, J. (2006). *Introduction to classical and modern test theory.* Kentucky: Cengage Learning.

Darrow, C. W. (1927). Sensory, secretory and electrical changes in the skin following bodily excitation. *The Journal of General Psychology, 10, 197-226.*

Darrow, C. W. (1929). Differences in the physiological reactions to sensory and ideational stimuli. *Psychological Bulletin, 50: 44-52.*

Darrow, C. W. (1934). The significance of skin resistance in the light of its relation to the amount of perspiration. *The Journal of General Psychology, 11, 451-452.*

Darrow, C. W. (1936). The galvanic skin reflex (sweating) and blood pressure as preparatory and facilitative functions. *Psychological Bulletin, 33, 73-94.*

Darrow, C. W. (1937). Neural mechanisms controlling the palmar galvanic skin reflex and palmar sweating: a consideration of available literature. *Archives of Neurology and Psychiatry, 37, 641-663.*

Darrow, C. W. (1964). The rationale for treating the change in galvanic skin response as a change in conductance. *Psychophysiology, 1, 31-38.*

Davis, R. C. (1953). Response and adaptation to brief noises of high intensity. *USN SAM Res. Rep., Contract AF 33(038)-19630.*

Davis, R. C. (1957). Response patterns. *Transactions of the New York Academy of Sciences, 19(8), 731-739.*

Davis, R. C., Buchwald, A. M., Frankman, R. W. (1955). Autonomic and muscular responses and their relation to simple stimuli. *Psychological Monographs, 69(20), 1-71.*

Dawkins, R. (2009). *The greatest show on earth: The evidence for evolution.* Great Britain: Bantam Press.

Dement, W. C. (1955). Dream recall and eye movement during sleep in schizophrenics and normal. *Journal of Nervous and Mental Diseases, 122, 263-269.*

Dement, W. C., & Kleitman, N. (1957a). Cyclic variations in EEG during sleep and their relation to eye movements, bodily motility and dreaming. *Journal of Electroencephalography and Clinical Neurophysiology, 9, 673-690.*

Dement, W. C., & Kleitman, N. (1957b). The relation of eye movements during sleep to dream activity: An objective method for the study of dreaming. *Journal of Experimental Psychology, 53, 339-346.*

Diner, B. C., Holcomb, P. J., & Dykman, R. A. (1985). P300 in major depressive disorder. *Psychiatry Research, 15, 175-184.*

Dykman, R. A. (1976). Conditioning as sensitization. *Pavlovian Journal of Biological Sciences, 2, 24-36.*

Dykman, R. A., Ackerman, Peggy T., Galbrecht, C. R., & Reese, W. G. (1963). Physiological reactivity to different stressors and methods of evaluation. *Psychosomaticedicine, 25, 37-50.*

Dykman, R. A., Corson, S. A., Reese, W. G., & Seager, L. D. (1962). Inhibition of urine flow as a component of the conditioned defense reaction. *Psychosomatic Medicine. Med., 24, 177-186.*

Dykman, R. A., & Gantt, W. H. (1959). The parasympathetic component of unlearned and cardiac responses. *Journal of Comparative and Physiological Psychology, 52, 163-167.*

Dykman, R. A., & Gantt, W. H. (1960). Experimental psychogenic hypertension: blood pressure conditioned to pain. *Johns Hopkins Bulletin, 107, 72-89.*

Dykman, R. A., Gantt, W. H., & Whitehorn, J. C. (1956). Conditioning as emotional sensitization and learning. *Psychology Monographs, 70 (Whole No. 422), 1-17.*

Dykman, R. A., Heimann, E. K., & Kerr, W. A. (1952). Lifetime worry patterns of three diverse adult cultural groups. *Journal of Social Psychology, 35, 91-100.*

Dykman, R. A., Reese, W. C., Galbrecht, C. R., & Thomasson, P. J. (1959). Psychophysiological reactions to novel stimuli: measurement, adaptation, and relationship of psychological and physiological variables in the normal human. *Annals of the New York Academy of Sciences, 79(3), 43-107.*

Dykman, R. A., & Shurrager, P. A. (1956). Successive and maintained conditioning in spinal carnivores. *Journal of Comparative and Physiological Psychology, 49, 27-35.*

Dykman, R. A., & Stalnaker, J. M. (1957). Survey of women physicians graduating from medical school 1925-1950. *Journal of Medical Education, 32, Part 2, 1-38.*

Edelberg, R. (1966). Response of cutaneous water barrier to ideational stimulation. *Journal of Comparative Physiology and Psychology, 61, 28-33.*

Edelberg, R., Wright, D. J. (1964). Two galvanic skin response effector organs and their stimulus specificity. Psychophysiology, 1, 39-47.

Foster, K. G., Weiner, J. S. (1970). Effects of cholinergic and adrenergic blocking agents on the activity of the eccrine sweat glands. *Journal of Physiology, 210, 883-895.*

Galbrecht, C. R., Dykman, R. A., Reese, W. G., & Suzuki, T. (1965). Intrasession adaptation and intersession extinction of the components of the orienting response. *Journal of Experimental Psychology, 70(6), 585-597.*

Gantt, W. H. (1944). *Experimental basis for neurotic behavior: Origin and development of artificially produced disturbances of behavior in dogs.* New York: Paul B. Hoeber, Inc.

Gantt, W. H. (1946). Cardiac conditioned reflexes to time. *Transactions of the American Neurological Association, 71(166).*

Gantt, W. H. (1953). Principles of nervous breakdown—schizokinesis and autokinesis. *Annals New York Academy of Sciences, 56, 143-163.*

Gisolfi, C. V., Robinson, S. (1970). Central and peripheral stimuli regulating sweating during intermittent work in men. *Journal of Applied Physiology, 29, 761-768.*

Gisolfi, C. V., Wenger, C. B. (1984). Temperature regulation during exercise: old concepts, new ideas. *Exercise and Sport Science Reviews, 12, 339-372.*

Haggard, E. A. (1949a). On the application of analysis of variance to GSR data: I. The selection of an appropriate measure. *Journal of Experimental Psychology, 39,378-392.*

Haggard, E. A. (1949b). On the application of analysis of variance to GSR data: II. Some effects of the use of inappropriate measures. *Journal of Experimental Psychology, 39, 861-867.*

Hall, K. J. (1997). *Carl Rogers.* Unpublished manuscript, Department of Psychology, Muskingum College, New Concord, Ohio.

Havighurst, R. J. (1972). *Developmental tasks and education.* London: Longman Group United Kingdom.

Haviland, W. A. (1994). *A Biological memoir of Wilton Marion Krogman.* Washington, D.C.: National Academy of Sciences.

Hilgard, E. R., & Marquis, D. G. (1940). *Conditioning and learning.* New York: Appleton.

Howe, E. S. (1958). GSR conditioning in anxiety states, normal, and chronic functional schizophrenic subjects. *The Journal of Abnormal and Social Psychology, 56(2), 183-189.*

Innes, I. R., & Nickerson, M. (1965). Drugs inhibiting the action of acetylcholine on structures innervated by postganglionic parasympathetic nerves. In Goodman, L. S., & Gilman, A. (Eds.), *The Pharmacological Basis of Therapeutics (3).* New York: Macmillan Co.

Johnson, L. C. (1963). Some attributes of spontaneous autonomic activity. *Journal of Comparative and Physiological Psychology, 56, 415-422.*

Joreskog, KG., & Sorbom, D. (1993). *LISREL 8 structural equation modeling with SMPLIS command language.* Hillsdale, NJ: Lawrence Erlbaum Associates Publishers.

Juniper, K. Jr., Blanton, D. E., & Dykman, R. A. (1967). Palmar skin resistance and sweat gland counts in drug and non-drug states. *Psychophysiology, 4, 231-243.*

Juniper, K. Jr., Dykman, R. A. (1967). Skin resistance, sweat-gland counts, salivary flow, and gastric secretion: Age, race, and sex differences, and intercorrelations. *Psychophysiology, 4, 216-222.*

Juniper, K. Jr., Stewart, JR., DeVaney, G. T., & Smith, T. J. (1964). Finger-tip sweat-gland activity and salivary secretion as indices of anticholinergic drug effect. *The American Journal of Digestive Diseases, 9, 31-42.*

Kellogg, W. N. (1946). A search for the spinal conditioned response. *American Psychologist, 1, 274-275.*

Kleitman, N. (1963). *Sleep and wakefulness.* Chicago: University of Chicago Press.

Kolka, M. A., & Stephenson, L. A. (1987). Cutaneous blood flow and local sweating after systemic atropine administration. *Pflugers Archiv, 410, 524-529.*

Kramer, M. (1994). The scientific study of dreaming. In M. H. Kryger, T. Roth, & W.C. Dement (Eds.), *Principles and Practice of Sleep Medicine, 2nd ed., (pp. 394-399)*. Philadelphia: Saunders.

Lacey, J. I. (1956). The evaluation of autonomic responses: toward a general solution. *Annals of New York Academy of Sciences, 67(5), 123-164.*

Lacey, J. I., Lacey, B. C. (1958a). Verification and extension of the principle of autonomic response stereotypy. *The American Journal of Psychology, 71, 50-73.*

Lacey, J. I., Lacey, B. C. (1958b). The relationship of resting autonomic activity to motor impulsivity. In H. C. Solomon, S. Cobb, & W. Pennfield (Eds.), *The Brain and Human Behavior.* Williams & Wilkins: Baltimore, MD.

Loney, J., & Milich, R. (1982). Hyperactivity, inattention, and aggression in clinical practice. In Wolraich, M. Routh DK, (Ed.), *Advances in developmental and behavioral pediatrics (pp. 68-69).*

Longmore, J., Jani, B., Bradshaw, C. M., Szabadi, E. (1986). Effect of locally administered anticholinesterase agents on the secretory response of human eccrine sweat glands to acetylcholine and carbachol. *British Journal of Clinical Pharmacology, 21, 131-135.*

Lorenz, K. (1950). The comparative method in studying innate behavior patterns. *Symposia of the Society for Experimental Biology, 4, 221-268.*

Low, J. O., Lunt, P. S., Srole, L., & Warner, L. W. (1963). *Yankee City.* Connecticut: Yale University Press.

MacIntyre, B. A., Bullard, R. W., Banerjee, M., Elizondo, R. (1968). Mechanism of enhancement of eccrine sweating by localized heating. *Journal of Applied Physiology, 25, 255-260.*

Marr, J. (2011). *The modifiers.* United States: Xlibris Publishing.

Matson, J.L. (1993) Handbook of Hyperactivity in Children. Allyn and Bacon, Boston, MA.

McGuigan, F. J., Ban, T. A. (Eds). (1987). *Monographs in psychobiology: An integrated approach. Critical issues in psychology, psychiatry, and physiology.* New York: Gordon and Breach Science Publishers.

Morgan, C. T. (1950). *Physiological psychology.* New York: McGraw Hill.

Nadal, E. R., Mitchell, J. W., Saltin, B., Stolwojk, J. A. J. (1971). Peripheral modifications to the central drive for sweating. *Journal of Applied Physiology, 31, 838-833.*

Nadal, E. R., Pandolf, K. B., Roberts, M. F., Stolwojk, J. A. J. (1974). Mechanisms of thermal acclimation to exercise and heat. *Journal of Applied Physiology, 37, 515-520.*

Pavlov, I. P. (1927). *Conditioned reflexes* (C. V. Anrep, Trans.). London and New York: Oxford University Press (Milford).

Pavlov, I. P. (1928). *Lectures on conditioned reflexes* (W. H. Gantt, Trans). New York: International Publishers.

Penny, D., L. R. Foulds, & M. D. Hendy. 1982. Testing the theory of evolution by comparing phylogenetic trees constructed from five different protein sequences. *Nature 297:197-200.*

Pivik. R. T. (2000). Sleep and dreaming. In J. Cacioppo, L. Tassinary, & G. Berntson (Eds.), *Handbook of Psychophysiology (pp. 687-716).* United Kingdom: Cambridge University Press.

Quinton, P. M. (1987). Physiology of sweat secretion. *Kidney International Supply Journal, 21, S102-S108.*

Rachman, S. (1960). Reliability of galvanic skin response measures. *Psychological Reports, 6, 326.*

Randall, W. C., Kimura, K. K. (1955). The pharmacology of sweating. *Pharmacology Reviews, 7, 365-397.*

Rescorla, R.A. (1967). Pavlovian conditions and its proper control procedures. *Psychology Review, 74, 71-80.*

Reese, W. G., Dykman, R. A., & Peters, J. E. (1987). Gantt on Gantt, In F. J. McGuigan, & T. A. Ban (Eds.), *Critical issues in psychology, psychiatry, and physiology (pp. 17-56).* New York: Gordon and Breach Science Publishers.

Robertshaw, D. (1975). In H. Blaschko, G. Sayers, & A. D. Smith, (Eds.), *Handbook of Physiology, vol VI, Endocrinology (pp. 591-603).* Washington, DC: American Physiological Society.

Rogers, C. (1942). *Counseling and psychotherapy.* Massachusetts: Houghton Mifflin Company.

Rogers, C. (1951). *Client-centered therapy.* Massachusetts: Houghton Mifflin Company.

Rogers. C. (1961). *On becoming a person.* Massachusetts: Houghton Mifflin Company.

Sacks, O. (1985). *The man who mistook his wife for a hat.* Austin, Texas: Touchstone.

Sato, K. (1977). The physiology, pharmacology, and biochemistry of the eccrine sweat gland. *Reviews of Physiology, Biochemistry, and Pharmacology, 79, 51-131.*

Shaywitz, SE. (1979). *Yale neuropsychoeducational assessment scales.* New Haven, CT: Yale University Press.

Sherrington, C. S. Sir. (1906). *The integrative action of the nervous system.* New York: C. Scribner's Sons.

Shibasaki, M., & Crandall, C. G. (2011). Mechanisms and controllers of eccrine sweating in humans. *Frontiers in Bioscience (Scholar Edition), 2,* 685–696.

Shurrager, P. S., & Dykman, R. A. (1951). Walking spinal carnivores. *Journal of Comparative and Physiological Psychology, 44, 252-262.*

Skinner, B. F. (1971). *Beyond freedom and dignity.* New York: Alfred A. Knopf, Inc.

Singer, J. D., & Willett, J. B. (2003). *Applied Longitudinal Data Analysis: Modeling Change and Event Occurrence.* New York: Oxford University Press.

Sokolov, E. N. (1960). Neuronal models and the orienting reflex. In Mary A.B. Brazier (Ed.), *The Central Nervous System and Behavior (pp. 187-276).* New York: Josiah Macy Jr. Foundation.

Sokolov, E. N. (1963). *Perception and the conditioned reflex.* Oxford: Pergamon Press.

Stevens, S. S. (1951). Mathematics, measurement and psychophysics. In S. S. Stevens, (Ed.), *Handbook of Experimental Psychology* (pp. 1-49). New York: Wiley.

Stevens, S. S., & Galanter, E. H. (1957). Ratio scales and category scales for a dozen perceptual continua. *Journal of Experimental Psychology, 54, 377-411.*

Taylor, J. (1953). A personality scale of manifest anxiety. *The Journal of Abnormal and Social Psychology, 48(2), 285-290.*

Tamhane, A. C., & Dunlop, D. D. (2000). *Statistics and data analysis: from elementary to intermediate.* Upper Saddle River, NJ: Prentice Hall.

Terman, L. M. (1916). *The measurement of intelligence.* Boston, Massachusetts: Houghton Mifflin Company.

Terman, L. M., & Merrill, M. A. (1937). *Measuring intelligence.* Boston, Massachusetts: Houghton Mifflin.

Terman, L. M., & Merrill, M. A. (1960). *Stanford-Binet Intelligence Scale: Manual for the Third Revision Form L-M.* Boston, Massachusetts: Houghton Mifflin.

Tinbergen, N. (1951). *The study of instinct.* Oxford: Clarendon Press.

Treffert, D. A. (2009). Savant syndrome: an extraordinary condition. A synopsis: past, present, and future. *Philosophical Transactions of the Royal Society B, 364, 1351-1357.*

Uno, H. (1977). Sympathetic innervation of the sweat glands and piloarrector muscles of macaques and human beings. *Journal of Investigative Dermatology, 69,112-120.*

Wada, M. (1950). Sudorific action of adrenalin on the human sweat glands and determination of their excitability. *Science, 111, 376-377.*

Webb, W. B. (1993). Dream theories of the ancient world. In M. A. Carskadon (Ed.), *Encyclopedia of Sleep and Dreaming (pp. 192-194).* New York: Macmillan.

Whitehorn, J. C. (1953). Introduction and survey of the problems of stress. In *Symposium on Stress.* Washington, D. C.: Army Medical Center Graduate School, Walter Reed Army Medical Center.

Wilson, J. D., & Dykman, R. A. (1960). Background autonomic activity in medical students. *Journal of Comparative and Physiological Psychology, 53(4), 405-411.*

Wilder, J. (1950). The law of initial value. *Psychosomatic Medicine, 12,* 392-400.

Wilder, J. (1957). The law of initial value in neurology and psychiatry: facts and problems. *Journal of Nervous Mental Diseases, 125, 73-86.*

Wittern, R. (1989). Sleep theories in antiquity and the Renaissance. In J. A. Horne (Ed.), *Sleep '88 (pp. 11-22).* Stuttgart: Fischer-Verlag.

Woodworth, R. S., & Schlosberg, H. (1954). *Experimental Psychology (Revised).* New York: Henry Holt and Company.

www.ingramcontent.com/pod-product-compliance
Lightning Source LLC
Chambersburg PA
CBHW070815180526
45168CB00002B/626